Blood, Sweat, & Years
Hack Your Body
A Guide For Peak Performance Living and Self Enlightenment

"The secrets to changing your physique, mind, and place in this world through exercise, nutrition, drugs, and meditation."

The objective of this book is to inform, educate, and entertain. It is not intended as a prescription or substitute for health care by a professional. I am not a doctor and recommend you seek professional guidance for any workout regimen or protocol you attempt in these pages.

"I was deep in the desert,
somewhere around Mt. Zion and the
Red Cliff's National Conservation Area.
I don't really know where exactly. I was kidnapped.
We were being stalked by a mountain lion and it was the
dead of night.
What saved us from being dinner was two Native American ghosts.
That's pretty much when it all started."

TABLE OF CONTENTS: 5
INTRODUCTION   8
Transformation   8
The Importance of Exercise for This   10
Journey   10
CHAPTER ONE   12
Epigenetics   12
Epigenetic Regulations of Metabolic Benefits Produced By Exercise
15
Exercise's Effects On Cancer   16
Exercising and the Aging Process   16
Exercise's Benefits on the Central Nervous System   17
CHAPTER TWO   18
Mysticism   18
Spirit Walkers   21
So What Is Mysticism?   28
CHAPTER THREE   31
Your Path   31
CHAPTER FOUR   39
Self Transcendence, Worshipping Yourself   39
CHAPTER FIVE   44
Take Back Control Of Your Life   44
CHAPTER SIX   47
Focus On The Present You 47
Take Inventory and Answer Some Questions 48
Identify The 4 Emotions That will Change Your Life: 50
FOUR Questions To Ask Yourself Right Now: 50
CHAPTER SEVEN 51
Why Are Experts Important?   51
Why Blood, Sweat, and Years?   52
CHAPTER EIGHT 61
Finding Your Passion   61
Setting Expectations   64
CHAPTER NINE   69
To Change Your Mind, Start with Your Body 69
Making The Commitment 71
CHAPTER TEN   74
Keys to Success   74
Taking Measurements   75

Fitness Trackers   76
Three Key Physical Measurements   77
Basal Metabolic Rate (BMR)   79
Lean Body Mass : LBM   80
Sterling-Pasmore (SLIGHTLY MODIFIED) 81
Basic Macronutrient Breakdowns: 86
Water   88
Salt / Sodium   90
Potassium   91
Why Do We Care About Water, Sodium, and Potassium?   92

CHAPTER TWELVE   93
The Importance of Maintaining A Healthy Bodyweight and BMI
93

CHAPTER THIRTEEN   98
Fasting 98

CHAPTER FOURTEEN   102
Carbohydrate Supercompensation   102
Sugar   106

CHAPTER FIFTEEN   108
Meditation - Bridging the Gap Between Mind and Body108

CHAPTER SIXTEEN   111
Crafting Your Routine   111
Exercise 111
Aerobic Exercise vs Anaerobic Exercise   112
Anaerobic Exercise   112
Aerobic Exercise 113
HIIT   114
Power Of The Heat : Training In The Heat   115

CHAPTER SEVENTEEN 119
Hot Yoga   119

CHAPTER EIGHTEEN   122
Manifesting   122

CHAPTER NINETEEN   124
Sleep and Sleep Hacking   124
Importance of Sleep   124
Sleep Hacking   126

CHAPTER TWENTY   128
Detoxification Diet Program   128

CHAPTER TWENTY ONE   131
Substances to Hack the Mind and Body   131
Caffeine 131

6

Cannabis132

How to use Cannabis - or Any Other Psychoactive Drug - Spiritually 136

Psilocybin and LSD for Depression 140

Anabolic and Androgenic Compounds   147

Testosterone   149

Deca Durabolin   153

Human Growth Hormone (HGH)   153

Clenbuterol Hydrochloride 155

Side effects of PED's   156

Restoring Natural Hormone Levels Post PED Use   157

CHAPTER TWENTY TWO   158

In Closing   158

INTRODUCTION
Transformation

"The path that does not run away from but embraces our suffering is the path that will lead us to liberation." Thich That Hanh

Weight loss, self enlightenment, when we get down to it, everyone is going to have a deeply personal and deeply unique experience when they decide to embark on this journey. Let's start with a word called self transformation. Self transformation is a fairly simple concept for everyone to grasp and you probably have your own definition, but let's wipe that slate clean for a second. Self transformation starts with the idea of one getting better at being oneself. Maybe you said to yourself one day, "I've had it! Enough is Enough." As far as I know, no one has ever said, "Hey! I'm going to go on this journey of becoming a miserable, horrible human." This book is going to totally disregard the idea of transforming into a negative human. It's about becoming the very best version of yourself that you can be.

So the idea starts at getting better. Whether or not you follow through, we can all agree where the starting point is. The idea of a better you. Once again this idea can be anything from getting a makeover, to deciding to lose weight, to buying a whole new wardrobe. Simple stuff. Easy to define.

Through this process of self examination, exploration, and ideally transformation, maybe even after a couple of failed attempts, or even when we succeed, we begin to examine, pretty much out of involuntary response, the reasons we wanted change in our life in the first place. That's the point when we start getting into a different word, self enlightenment. Looking for those deeper truths. Our job and something we are going to talk about in this book is how to connect the mind and the body. A fully functional human needs to have their mind and their body on the same level of being in shape. One way we are going to achieve that synergy is

8

through strenuous physical exercise. Physically pushing ourselves to the limit is a proven method of quieting down the outside world and connecting us to that inner dialogue that we have been having trouble hearing. We will be discussing, fairly in depth, how to connect the mind and the body, as well as how to have an optimally trained machine.

As a body hacker we are engaged in altering our system features to accomplish a goal that differs from the original purpose of the system. Hacking's definition refers to non-malicious activities involving unusual or improvised alterations to equipment, processes, and systems and that is what we are doing to achieve our goals.

Once we have had a few successful positive habit changes in our life, maybe created some positive daily rituals, we begin to start looking inward on a consistent basis. It usually happens naturally as working out, walking, and being strict on our diet can force us into a meditative state just out of those things becoming routine. Maybe we begin looking at our spirituality or our religious beliefs. Maybe beginning to see patterns that emerge consistently throughout our lives. Maybe just realizing you were never really happy all along and are finally getting a taste of what you think that happiness is.

If we accomplish just one goal like weight loss, changing jobs, breaking up with that not so special person, we then have an opportunity, a fresh start, to begin creating who we really are. Rock bottom is a beautiful place that most people never get to experience. It's really the only place, besides your funeral, where you get to see who your friends are, who loves you, and who is willing to stick around through the hard times. The true way to find out who you really are and what you like is to try and experience as much as you can, all the time. Just think of trying to achieve strategic sensory overload as much as possible. "How ya gonna know you don't like anchovies if you don't eat an anchovy?" Right?

Many of the lessons and theories in this book come from autodidactic means, but that does not mean they are not based in substance. There are a lot of stories about me growing up. In the end, these stories fit into my narrative and they all make sense. It's real and it's relevant. I would also be doing a disservice to the memory of the many people who are in this book, many of whom are not alive anymore, if I didn't honor what they have meant to me. This book is packed and I mean packed with information that will bring you up to speed with where self enlightenment can go, where physique building and athletic performance can collide, how to safely explore your mind, and how to safely push your body to new levels.

I implore you to read this book with an open mind, always remembering that you can do whatever you want with your life. There is a lot of science in this book, but there is also a lot of pseudo science because I believe it's important to think outside the box. Science doesn't explain everything and not one person is the same in their physical and mental journey. Diet and exercise should not be set in stone and spirituality allows us a little leeway to interpret for our needs.

My goal is to give you as much information that I can in the clearest presentation possible. After you are done you will be able to create a spiritual and physical journey that will bring happiness and abundance for you, however you choose to attack it. With that said, we are going start with what I think is the most important part of a spiritual journey and that is exercise.

The Importance of Exercise for This Journey

65 billion years ago when humans first started walking the planet (the oldest remains of modern day humans, found in Morocco in 2017, go back roughly 315,000 years) they weren't sitting in cubicles, in little productivity farms called cities,

where they would go home at night to watch the wall. Humans were roaming the earth sometimes for days at a time, looking for food or for other humans to fuck or kill. The need for strenuous physical exercise is encoded into the human genome and is a natural remedy for nearly all that ails you both mentally, physically, and spiritually. If you tell yourself you are sick, you will be sick forever.

Physical exercise contributes to a better quality of life via the changes that it causes in the functioning of various physiological systems. (The changes it causes in your body.) This book is going to discuss the science and pseudo science of hacking your body and reaching whatever type of enlightenment you seek. It's not a prescription and I am in no way a doctor. It's a blueprint to a way of life. In the end, diet and nutrition are really just about numbers and staying consistent. That's the secret and we are going to decode what it takes to get to the next level.

CHAPTER ONE
Epigenetics

Epigenetics is the study of gene expression. Epigenetic alterations, induced by the good stress of physical exercise, have a positive impact on a multitude of biological functions. Our goal is to learn how to manipulate the body so that we can increase the efficiency and change how many of the systems in our body work. Exercise has been proven not only to improve physical health, but mental health as well. Our program utilizes the stress from strenuous exercise to access the mind.

To get a little deeper into it and to give you the scientific definition, epigenetics is the study of the changes in phenotype, which is an observable physical or biochemical change in an organism, namely us, without a change in genotype, which is the genetic code and carries all the genetic information.

An example would be changing the speed of our metabolism by applying outside forces of planned nutrition and HIIT (high intensity interval training) exercises. The end result causes a body to activate genes in order to adapt to the new energy demands that are being applied. However, you stay human and don't become an alien or grow a third arm because you were using a bigger dumbbell. Your underlying code is the same; you just have new adaptations going on within the body. Gene = Code. We are hacking code.

For the purpose of accomplishing our goals, we will be manipulating (hacking) our physical and mental environment using nutrition, exercise, meditation, and if you choose, drugs, to activate genes that were not being expressed previously. The body has the ability to adapt, change, and heal at a substantially faster rate when given the proper stimulus and basic building blocks.

So why is epigenetics important? I bring it up because the body is forever in a constant state of cell death and rebirth.

By turning on certain genes in our body we can ensure that when the new cells are reproduced from the old ones that the new gene expressions are carried over. A study published in the U.S. National Library of Medicine reported, "That if one chooses to compare the number of bacteria in the human body to the number of nucleated human cells, the ratio will be about 10:1."

At the end of the day we are technically more bacteria than human and all of this plays a role on us at the end of the day. It's not just little Joey up in his head. It's trillions upon trillions of human cells and bacteria all molding into this thing we call a human and creating something we think is a consciousness.

There is a popular belief that your body completely turns all of its cells over every seven years. It has actually been proven that different parts of the body regenerate at different rates.

Your liver is replaced roughly every 300 to 500 days. So if you are a heavy drinker think about what going cold turkey for a year could do for you. You would have essentially a new liver in give or take a year.

Your intestines are new every 16 years, but their lining every five days. So theorctically, it will take a long time to repair your gut, but if you are having immediate problems you can make some adjustments and in five days will know if you have produced any benefits. Your red blood cells are replaced every 120 days. Your skin every 39-40 days and your skeleton is replaced every ten years. That's what small positive changes in your life are going to add up to over the short and the long term.

Epigentics plays a critical part in gene expression and regulation. When a gene expresses itself that means it "turns on." Scientists are still debating how many cells are actually in the human body, but the estimation is between 30 and 40 trillion cells. Nonetheless, It's an inconceivable number. Not to mention that there is an untold amount of trillions of bacterial cells living within you as well. All of these things playing a factor on who you are.

During your lifetime, only a fraction of the genes that each cell carries will be expressed. Throughout our lifetime our genes are turned on and off. In development, one cell expresses to look like a liver, the other an eyeball. Gene regulation is critical for life and allows the body to quickly adapt to its environment. Hence the theory that you can selectively turn on genes by applying specific stresses to the body. In our case, exercise and nutrition stresses will be applied.

I bring this up because when I was lazy, fat, and unmotivated, it wasn't until I started applying different stresses, primarily physical, to my body that it was forced to change. I didn't know what epigenetics was at the time, I just knew that the body is an adaptation machine and will adapt to most stresses that are thrown at it.

Just a few examples from my life: my metabolism went from exclusively storing fat to burning fat. Through vigorous exercise, I began wanting to push myself further, forcing me to clean up my diet and allowing me to lose 100 pounds. And through making small adjustments and accomplishing small goals, I have achieved a better overall mental and physical state of being. It finally feels good to be in my skin. No longer do I eat a piece of cake and gain ten pounds. No longer are my immediate thoughts in the morning negative. It all happened because I changed the expressions being presented. I had to change my life. I had to exercise in order to do this.

Gene regulation refers to the mechanisms that act to induce or repress the expression of a gene. Gene regulation is produced, in our case, by changing how we eat, what we think,

AND adding vigorous exercise over a prolonged period of time.[1]

Although our genetic makeup is more stable during adulthood, scientist agree that it is still dynamic and modifiable by lifestyle choices and environmental influence. Research is now suggesting that it is becoming more apparent that epigenetic effects occur not just in the womb, but over the full course of a human life. There are numerous examples of epigenetics that show how different lifestyle choices and environmental exposures can alter marks on top of DNA and play a role in determining health outcomes. Here are a few examples to drive home the point.

Epigenetic Regulations of Metabolic Benefits Produced By Exercise

It is well established that physical exercise causes alterations in the expression of human skeletal muscle genes, as a mechanism of adaptation not only to the mechanical load but also to the metabolic stress of exercise. Many of those changes in gene expression can occur through epigenetic regulations which are induced by exercise and are related to metabolic processes.

Specifically, high intensity exercise (HIIT, see HIIT section) causes a reduction in a specific group of gene expressions that are related to numerous diseases including obesity, diabetes, atherosclerosis, and cancer. Endurance exercise has been shown to alter the expression of various types of genes which play a key role in the maintenance of skeletal muscle mass as well.

---

[1]"Can genes be turned on and off in cells?" National Institutes of Health, U.S. National Library of Medicine. https://ghr.nlm.nih.gov/primer/howgeneswork/geneonoff (7/1/2018).

Exercise's Effects On Cancer

Physical activity is currently suggested as a protective factor against cancer, which may lower the risk of cancer occurrence and mortality. The Mayo Clinic states that, "The protective role of exercise is noted in many cancers, including lung, endometrial, colon and prostate." In fact, "Studies show there's a 25 percent reduction in the risk of breast cancer among the most physically active women, compared to those who are least active."[2]

Another underlying mechanism for cancer is chronic inflammation that can be mediated through exercise. Yes, physical exercise can make us sore through the release of lactic acid and other regulatory chemicals, but it also activates the natural anti-inflammatory responses throughout the body. And this has an overall net positive effect for the body.

Exercising and the Aging Process

Age related diseases such as rheumatoid arthritis, atherosclerosis, and type II diabetes are all associated with chronic inflammation. Religious adherence to an exercise program reduces the expression of pro inflammatory chemicals through epigenetic modifications, therefore preventing many inflammatory diseases.

Lastly, although aging is usually related to increased frailty as a result of the aging of muscles, exercise regulates the genes which control the rate at which your muscles shrink (atrophy) and regrow.

---

[2] Dorfner, Micah. "Keep Moving: The Importance of Exercise in Cancer Survivorship." Mayo Clinic. http://www.bibme.org/citation-guide/chicago/website/ (7/1/2018).

Exercise's Benefits on the Central Nervous System

Exercise plays an important role on brain cognition throughout our lifetime, but especially as we begin to age. Strenuous exercise has been contributed to the promotion of mental health and resistance to neurological disorders and brain syndromes thought the aging process. A few disorders that have had various studies performed on them with great success would include Alzheimer's, depression, manic episodes, bipolar disorder, REM sleep deprivation, and attention deficit hyperactivity disorder (ADHD). [3]

[3] Ntanasis-Stathopoulous, J., Tzanninis, J-G., Philippou, A., Koutsilieris, M. "Epigenetic regulation on gene expression induced by physical exercise." Department of Experimental Physiology, Medical School, National and Kapodistrian University of Athens, Athens, Greece. https://www.researchgate.net/publication 237004244_Epigenetic_regulation_on_gene_expression_induced_by_physical_exercise (5/7/2018).

CHAPTER TWO
Mysticism

Spiritually, enlightenment, searching for the deeper truths, it all falls under the same umbrella to me and that is one that leads to mysticism. Even as I sit here typing this out, struggling to breathe with my 40 pound dog on my lap, I have an overwhelming feeling of déjà vu, that I have been here or done this a million times before. Maybe not me, but one of my timelines has definitely sat here had this same experience.

I grew up Roman Catholic, went to grammar school where we had chapel every morning, and in high school, after being arrested for smoking a joint on the street (this was the '90s), got sent to a rehabilitation program in the Utah desert where I had my mind blown. I eventually attended a Catholic college in Connecticut, but along the way lost interest in practicing organized religion and stopped caring for traditional methods of worship. It took years before I got my shit together and really started trying to make sense of it all.

Rewind, rewind, rewind. Back to the desert. We are about three weeks in. I was slow to get with the program. The average attendee in wilderness school is there for roughly 30 days. I was there for 92. Once I decided the only way out was to play the game and get with the program, I quickly rose from the single laziest out of shape human in the group to one of the group leaders. I have always had a problem with motivation, getting started, but once I get in the groove one of my superpowers is that I can concentrate intensely on anything like it is the only thing that exists for long periods of time.

I'm a numbers guy now, but when I was a teenager I was not. At the wilderness school I was sent to you would get a number. This number was essentially based on your rank in the group or how long you have been in the group and after the rough initial few weeks I went to number one.

Numbers were given so that the wilderness counselor could keep track of every kid in the program. If you took a shit and went out of eyesight, you called out your number the entire time. It didn't matter if it was day or night. If you were out of eyesight, you called your number continuously until you came back from using the latrine, getting wood, whatever.

The group I was in was a mixed hodgepodge. We cleverly named ourselves the Lone Wolves. We were put together out of a mess of other groups and a polliwog camp (when you first arrive you are a polliwog). Among the guys I learned to trust the most during my time in the desert was a guy from Utah also named Joe who was a little older than I was and was there for smoking meth. Coincidentally, he also knew what cactuses and mushrooms to eat in the desert. Another kid, 13, named JB, there for using acid, was my friend throughout my entire time there. Both of these guys were cool and both were dead by the time I was in college.

Due to a recent graduation, many of the groups were being combined. It seemed like they were trying to motivate the lazier groups by merging them with mine. An all girls group, known to move literally zero miles per day, was added to our group. One of the girls we quickly dubbed the "green goblin" because she caused so many problems and was difficult to look at. There was a specific incident involving her. We were out of water and it had been a few days since we had seen a watering hole, or any water for that matter. We were hiking between five to ten miles a day, depending on the terrain. The green goblin on day three of no water, on a day where the counselors had stated it was imperative to find water, well, on that day she decided to do a sit in.

Stories like this are funny to me because, although the group did not have water, a few smart people did. When first checked into the program, each person was given a gasoline container which held a gallon of water, along with two Nal-gene bottles. A gallon of water weighs roughly 8.5 pounds, then add two Nalgene's. I learned very early on, right around my second week when I ran out of water, that water was the most important resource we had in the desert.

Water is relatively heavy, and it's a 100% necessity whether you are in a survival situation or not. We happened to be in one. With that being said, a lot of people in our group were known to pour out their water so that they would have lighter packs, depending on the stronger ones in the group to share when they ran out. But this game had become tiring and it was usually the dudes with the water.

I carried around 20 pounds of water, scoring an extra gas tank from a graduating group member. The total amount of water I carried in my pack was 2.25 gallons. My philosophy still to this day is that the weight difference between a 70 pound pack, then adding one more gallon and ending up with a 78.5 pound pack is negligible after you have been carrying it around for a month or so. Water in the desert is essential. It's literally your gas tank to life.

JB and the other Joe were on the same page. We all carried around a lot of water and felt that it wasn't our job to keep this people alive. In the end, it was really only the lazy girl group and the goblin who didn't have water. The counselors knew this, but for some reason they still seemed to take immense pleasure out of not telling the entire group. When the goblin made it clear that she was not moving and could care less if we all died of dehydration, they put her in a headlock and dragged her for at least 300 yards until she gave up and got with the program. To the green goblins credit she fought like a wild animal caught in a cargo net right after a trap has sprung. It just wasn't enough to battle the two adult male counselors.

In my wilderness school if people's lives were on the line they would resort to force for the greater good of the group. Remember this was the 90s and you could get away with it. You could never get away with some of the tactics that were used back then today as society is much softer. Twenty years ago humans were just tougher.

Spirit Walkers

Night hiking was not an optimal thing for the group to do unless we had a full moon or close to it. At night in the desert, the temperature drops, it's harder to see unless there is a ton of moonlight, and, believe it or not, there are many predators lurking around. Occasionally we would take a night hike that was beautiful and not really planned.

On one particular night hike we knew that there was another group up the gully at a camp we had stayed at a few days prior. We decided to do what was known as a coo.

A coo in desert rehab is when you sneak up on another group in the night, hide in the bushes, then leap out and scare the shit out them. Cheap sober thrills.

My group, the Lone Wolves were staying in a very special location. We had set ourselves up for the past few days at a camp that had river with fresh fish running through it year round, a hot spring, and the only greenery available for miles. To get to it was a treacherous hike down a dried up riverbed that was known to flash flood. That dry bed eventually led to a cliff and if you were brave enough maneuver your way down the side of it you were in an oasis in the middle of nowhere.

I was in this wilderness program for 92 days and this was a camp was one we hit a few times, maybe three or four during my stay. Here we could wash ourselves in the hot spring, fish, and usually would stay for for 2 or 3 days at a time due to the rough hike in. That is basically the only excuse to stay at the camp longer than a day as the counselors always had us on the move. It was also one of the only places in the desert were it was lush with greenery year round. Anyway, the coo.

We break camp and head to do our coo. Or hike out of the dry river bed as I mentioned before was a rough one and eventually it leads us to the salt basin where we had stayed a few nights before. I clearly remember the night because of how windy it was. It was one of those eerily windy nights where you feel like you are being watched or there are spirits in the air. I'm sure you've had one experience at least where the wind blows and the hair stands up on the back of your neck. That was the entire night.

Off the salty basin was a mirage of sorts. There was a burnt out barn and down the hill behind it was a field of hot dog grass basically growing in a swamp. I remember the camp well because next to the swamp was a real patch of grass half the size of a football field where we slept out in the open on our tarps two or three times in the past.

I also refer to this camp as willow camp. As a city boy, I didn't know what hot dog grass or cattail grass was. I really thought willows, actually small shrubs, were the same thing at the time. We quickly labeled the willow camp as haunted because weird things would happen. For example, it could be a beautiful night, you could be dead asleep under the stars on top of a tarp, and boom! Lightning hits relatively close to you and you gotta make shelter. Also, the burnt out barn was very random in the middle of nowhere.

My first real experience of some mind blowing and, at this point I would call it spiritual shit that I can't explain, was that night. Willow camp was, for sure, spiritually charged, and every time we were there something crazy and unexplainable would happen. It's because of this night I started questioning everything and believing in spirits and in mother nature as the root of it all.

The weirdness started in the hot dog grass. Our group had set up camp for the night in the flats. We had just done a night hike and the coo was going to be done with no packs. This was our second or third time time sleeping in the flats. Nothing weird had ever happened at that location - yet.

After we hit the flats. We walked for what felt like forever. At some point, maybe 30 to 40 minutes, we could see the burnt out barn shell. Down the hill about 75 to 100 yards, was the field and to the left of it was the tall swamp grass. We headed for the hot dog grass. To do the coo we would would have to go left before the barn cutting through the swamp.

The entire group was in the swamp moving slowly. Coos are meant to raise group moral, to bond and were supposed to be fun. Walking through the swamp, we were huddled very close together like soldiers. Our counselor gave us the sign to pause, raising his fist in the air like we were in the military. Everyone was dead quiet. Along with JB and Joe, the group leaders at the time, we moved up to the front where our counselor was peeking through the grass. All of a sudden, we hear something breaking the hot dog grass branches roughly 15 to 20 yards behind the group. I start to think, "Can we be getting reversed cooed?" We shake it off and move ahead.

So the plan goes off without a hitch, our group making enough strange noises in the bushes, throwing rocks in random directions, terrifying our peers, and eventually we all run out and have a good laugh around the camp fire. When we finally left for the trek back to camp, it was late.
An hour later, we are still not back at camp. It's windy. It's cold. The fun is over and it's time for bed. Joe and I were at the front of the pack when we decided to stop and get our bearings. For some reason and, at the same time, we both looked to the left. In the sage bushes, about ten feet from us, flashed two beady yellow green eyes. I blinked and said to Joe, "Yo, what the fuck was that?" I started to walk over to see what it was and found that we were standing in our camp.

That's how dark it was that night. We shrugged off the beady little eyes and everyone hits the sack.

That night it was so fucking cold. It was windy and it was one of those nights where you cinch up the sleeping bag and you just have your nose come out of the hole. In wilderness, you don't actually sleep in a tent. You sleep in A-frames or whatever else you choose to build that is made out of your tarp. You connect the tarps with a rock that is rolled into two separate tarp corners called a "Deadman." The tarp is also what you use to make a burrito for your hiking pack.

I can remember it like it was yesterday. Although it's not scary now, it was incredibly scary back then and still to this day I can only half explain what happened. I don't know how long I had been asleep, but it must have been for an hour or so because at this point I was less cinched and my eyes and nose were exposed to the cold. From the middle of a dead sleep I woke up with a feeling I had never had before. More terrified and afraid for my life than I had ever been. Terrified to the point where I couldn't even blink, move, or scream for help. All I could do was keep looking at the ceiling of the tent knowing that I was being watched and possibly was about to die. Even as I write this, the hairs on my neck are starting to shift in confusion.

Finally after what felt like an eternity, I mustered up the courage to strain my eyes as far as I could towards the entrance of the tent on the right, only barely moving my neck as I was for sure I was dead if I did. At the entrance of the tent, I saw an elderly Native American couple, not like the ones you see stereotyped on old television shows wearing feather head dresses, but a modern old Indian couple. The man had a red plaid worker type jacket on, peering into the entrance from the left side of the opening. I remember breathing a sigh of relief, like I am at this moment, and going back to sleep.

The next morning our counselor, Jay, woke me up before any other of the campers. He took me outside the tent and asked me about the eyes I had mentioned on our hike back. He showed me a circle of paw prints around our tent and told me that a mountain lion must have been stalking us all night.

I went back inside the shelter and got ready to prepare my breakfast. I couldn't help but to keep on thinking that all those noises we heard in the swamp, all the other creep shit that was happening that night, me waking up, almost shitting myself, that there was no doubt in my mind, we were stalked by a mountain lion. We were also visited by something else. (However it's impossible to prove that my mind wasn't playing tricks on me in a moment of fight or flight.) It was clear to both me and my counselor that we had both gotten lucky that night.

I don't know if the Indian couple was protecting all of us or just me, or if it was even real. It could have been human spirits that were attached to that particular mountain lion. I'll never know. What I do know is that night and many others out in the desert were unexplainable. And that's why it's so important to get back to that.

After the mountain lion experience, as far as I was concerned, church was the same book every year. Year in and year out, it started with Christmas, even though that's not where it starts. And though I couldn't explain what happened in the desert, for me it was real. I understood then and understand now that when I read about ancient cultures worshipping the sun or the moon or an animal, those practices don't seem so far fetched. Those are idols you can actually experience. For all I know if I had seen those footprints outside my tent 500 years ago and understood that the animal had spared me that night? I might have started to worship the mountain lion.

Life is ever changing; organized religion doesn't and in general religion doesn't have a great track record overall, not just now, but throughout history. Also, our own personal lives change virtually every day. Right around my sophomore year of high school, one of my best friends was killed by a drunk driver in a car accident. I began really questioning the guy upstairs and what it was all about. Remember wilderness. After going to Catholic grammar school and having to wake up on a Sunday to go to church while God rested, getting sent to the desert, character education school, and then having my best friend die… I was pretty much over the whole praying to God thing.

I'm not anti organized religion by any means, and people can do whatever they want to do. It's just that by the end of my 20's I had already traveled some of the world, got sent to a few places people don't want to get sent to, done a few things people don't ever want to do, lost a few friends, and made it out alive.

By the end of my 20's and early 30's, I had also lost all of my grandparents, multiple acquaintances, an ex girlfriend, and two of my best friends. I couldn't understand, and even have had tarot card readers ask me why death continuously follows or followed me around. I've had a few close calls myself and that is the most unexplainable part, how I made it and so many others didn't. Those losses have helped me to realize that everyday needs to be lived like your last.

I've always felt that praying didn't do much for me. At best I would call it wishful thinking when I apply it. However, it does work for some people like my mom, one of the main reasons I am named after St. Joseph. I think in order for praying to truly work that you must be a true, and I mean true, believer. In fact, for anything to work you have to be a true believer.

I know a very close personal family friend. She has lost literally every single one of her eight brothers and sisters, has a debilitating chronic disease, lost her husband, and her daughter passed away under suspicious circumstances. She still goes to church every Sunday and thanks God for being alive. I couldn't do it. For a while I started to tell myself that shit just happens, and to a degree it does, but that is not a positive way to operate in life, as a pedestrian, an onlooker, or just a witness.

Oddly enough, at the same time, whenever I am in my most dire moments of need, I find myself asking God for help out of an involuntary response. I think everyone does that, shoots from the hip. It's still hard for me to believe that that is a "Wizard of Oz" or one dude pulling the stings up there. I have also been in two major car accidents where the occupants should have died. In both cases, the car was totaled. Unfortunately for some, I'm still here pissing people off. How tripped out is that?

On the flip side of organized religion, my grandmother who was respectful of the church, but always weary of priests' intentions, was a straight up Italian witch. She would practice something called The Evil Eye or as she would call it Malocchio. Whenever I would get sick or have a problem in life, she would fill up the sink in the kitchen, start speaking in tongue, spritzing olive oil in the water, burning matches. I remember her telling me one time that someone was collecting my footsteps. Her juju worked every time.

Even as I research this I remember her pouring the olive oil into the water, speaking her prayers and spells, making signs of the cross from time to time and looking to see if the oil would separate or stay together. This was how she would break a curse or a sickness. Or whatever she deemed I had. Malocchio can only be practiced by women and only learned on Christmas Eve. This is something I would have loved to have learned would I have been allowed. People don't get to experience that old world magic anymore. My aunt is trained, however, there is no one interested who is female to learn it in my family. In today's society, people don't get to learn stuff life that anymore. We are too far removed from our roots.

Church, Italian witchcraft, the occult, self worship, body hacking it's all very interesting stuff. What's really interesting is the idea that most of the ancient religions we typically think about today are probably just made up, or based off the true story.

For example I can go to the Metropolitan Museum of Art in Manhattan and see Egyptian artifacts. I can see Mayan ruins and ancient Japanese temples, but I can't go to the Met and see Jesus' slippers, his cross, his grail, or anything at all. Even at the Vatican we have to resort to the Sistine Chapel or a statue as a reference to the Bible.

We don't have Adam's remains or a petrified apple next to some snake skin. I'm not specifically singling out the Catholic faith, although it might seem that way. It is just the religion I am most familiar with as it is how I was raised and was the denomination of schools I attended for the majority of my life. What I am trying to do is show you that many of the major religions are lacking in facts. Even the Bible Lands Museum in Jerusalem only has some inscriptions on limestone, some tablets, a couple random sarcophaguses, but does not have Moses' bones or relics of Noah's Ark. This is where things like faith come into play to help fill in the gaps.

So What Is Mysticism?

According to Evelyn Underhill, mysticism is "the science or art of the spiritual life."[1] Also, "Mysticism would best be thought of as a constellation of distinctive practices, dis-

---

[1] Underhill, Evelyn. "Mysticism: A Study in the Nature and Development of Spiritual Consciousness." Originally published, 1911. Reissued, Dover Pubications, March 12, 2002. (6/14/2018)

courses, texts, institutions, traditions, and experiences aimed at human transformation." [2]

"The first time I ever gave thought to being a mystic or what mysticism actually was occurred when I was on a yoga retreat in Hawaii in 2018. I had always been a spiritual person, but I didn't have a word for it. I first heard the term when during a conversation the group of people I was hanging out with referred to me as a learned mystic and to another person in the group as a natural mystic. It wasn't until months later that I sat down and tried to figure out what made someone a learned mystic as opposed to a natural mystic. I believe the only difference is that the learned mystic has to be turned on to the way they should have been operating all along, while the natural mystic is that way from an early age. The learned mystic was always a mystic (a true mystic), they were just not in touch with their true self.

Mysticism is defined as the practice of religious ecstasies. Religious ecstasies being defined as a type of altered state of consciousness characterized by greatly reduced external awareness and expanded interior mental and spiritual awareness, sometimes accompanied by visions and frequently promoting strong emotional and physical euphoria. Any religion is capable of experiencing religious ecstasies. Yoga, not a religion but a proven method in obtaining both reduced external awareness and internal clarity, is also proven to produce those feelings of euphoria that we are seeking.

Mysticism also has a fairly broad definition. William James a deceased American philosopher and psychologist tried to narrow it down for us a little bit by stating, "In mystic states we

---

[2] Gellman, Jerome. "Mysticism." The Stanford Encyclopedia of Philosophy (Summer 2011 Edition). Edward N. Zalta (ed.) plato.stanford.edu. https://plato.stanford.edu/entries/mysticism/ (Accessed date).

both become one with the Absolute and we become aware of our oneness."

Another thing to note is you don't have to be a mystic or be associated with mysticism to have a mystical experience. Everyone is capable of of having experiences which are intense, integrating, self-authenticating, and liberating.

Shamanism, which is a practice that involves reaching an altered states of consciousness in order to interact with a spirit or sprit world, channels transcendental energies into this world and is another form of mysticism. Often times in Shamanism substances like ayahuasca, mescaline, or psilocybin mushrooms will be used in the ritual as well. Shamans are considered the link between the human plane and plane of the spirit world. To a place of higher existence. They link to the spirit world in order to heal, contact deceased ancestors, influence the weather, and uplift consciousness.

For mystics the entire world is connected. They believe all living things have a spirit even things that are not living, like the earth and the ocean.

CHAPTER THREE
Your Path

"Honor yourself. Worship yourself. Meditate on yourself. God dwells within you as you." Swami Muktananda

There is a subject that is almost unfathomable and barely possible to comprehend for those who have not yet had their breakthrough revelation, had a near death experience, hit rock bottom, or lost someone close to them. It's that tomorrow is not guaranteed. If you are reading this it is because you seek to experience life and all its mysteries above anything else.

It is the realization that true living can only be lived in a space that moves with the current of the universe. For lack of a better term "going with the flow." Spiritual truths cannot be understood by intellect or, for that matter, be correctly identified or defined by words. Experience is the only thing that brings us to understanding.

In today's technology-addicted society, there is an ever present realization and need for the consumption of a product called enlightenment. Humans are yearning for a new level of self-awareness at a faster rate than ever before. People are beginning to feel the need to connect. Maybe it's because we are more detached from who we are than ever before? It used to be that we escaped the real world by going on the internet. Now it seems people are yearning to escape the internet by going back to the real world. I applaud everyone who is in that boat.

If you are reaching moments in your life or believing that you need a fundamental shift in consciousness, or just that a change must be made, you don't have to navigate it alone. Buddha was recorded as saying,

"Our suffering needs to be identified… That the wounds in our heart need to become the obsession of our meditations."

At this point you might not even know what your suffering is, but at least you have taken the first step on your journey toward self betterment.

Let the truths you are are seeking about yourself be unfathomable to those who have not yet had their "moment," always being mindful of your awareness helping others to grow in the process.

Spirituality has always been more interesting to me than religion. Growing up, I attended Catholic grammar school, K-8, where every day began with chapel. I went to church every Sunday and then attended a Catholic college in Connecticut where I studied business. I became obsessed with the thought of success over anything else, even happiness. Money became my definition of success.

I graduated in 2006 and it seemed like every year after that I always stepped in some short of shit, meaning a good job, a strong financial agreement, awesome prospects, but as the years went by the opportunities got less and less and I always seemed to fuck up the good ones. It wasn't until about 2012, when I weighed 273 pounds, eating five to seven Percocets and a Xanax bar a day, that I had my moment. My first of many self aware "holy shit" moments over the past ten years that have led me to write this book.

My spark for weight loss change happened one day at work. I was walking down the underground hallway of a major casino hotel where I worked on my way to lunch at the cafeteria with friends when my calves cramped up. I could literally no longer move my legs one inch further.

Under the hotels of Las Vegas are miles of tunnels. The walk to lunch which we so lovingly nicknamed "The I-15" (named after the local freeway), was about 200 yards away from the front desk area where we worked. At about 100 yards into the walk, I was done. My legs felt as though they were stuck in cement. Pretending to get a phone call and telling my peers to walk ahead of me, I started to freak out until the pain subsided. I'm sure my ass was sweating through my suit pants as well.

A few months after that I quit my job. At the time I was making roughly 8k-10k a month. Not a huge sum of money, but not a normal salary for a front desk agent. It just so happened that I worked for the best hotel in the world and made a a lot of money for them in the process.

The truth of the matter is I quit because of a chip on my shoulder. I had gotten suspended on a guest complaint (this is no big surprise if you know me), but this complaint was actually unwarranted and the suspension was getting drawn out. So being on lots of drugs, being unhappy about my weight, myself in general and thinking that it was easy to get bags of money like that, I quit. In the end it was the best thing that I ever did. However…

I was used to living like a king. My ritual for the weekend was poker or the club and, if you asked me twice, craps with a large buy in. I would drink as much as I could and play until I had smoked enough cigarettes, eaten enough pills, and found some tourist to try and get sleazy with. My nights usually ended in fast food and lots of pot smoking.

So when I semi-retired, out of really just being young and not knowing how good I had it, I decided to focus on losing weight. I made it my obsession. I read everything I could get my hands on. I experimented with every diet. I starved myself and I hired many experts to learn from. I also needed to keep making money. So drug dealing sounded like a good idea. Specifically, weed.

During this period of time cannabis was in a super gray area in the state I was living in, what popular culture calls the black market, but I call the regular market and the market was thriving. I had blown through my bank account. I had cashed out my 401k and I had about ten grand left to my name. I was still spending at the old income rate so I sat my roommate down at the time, a tired, depressed old grouch of a loser poker player, who we will call Snake, and I told him the plan. We were going to call a friend of mine in California take five thousand of my dollars, get as much as we could on credit, and we were going to start selling weed immediately. Credit is just what it sounds like. You get to take product for nothing upfront for a higher agreed price for later payment. It's crazy because as I was getting into the business I knew what the prices in New York were like for pounds, but had no idea what things went for on the West Coast. Snake had nothing going on so he agreed and we were off to California.

So my "friend" who was supposed to help us out didn't actually come through on the first run, but instead put us in touch with this middle aged hippy lady named Christmas, who lived on the beach in Malibu. I learned very quickly that there are no real friends in the game. Christmas was a real life Nancy Botwin, played by Mary-Louise Parker on Showtime's *Weeds*. We met in a 1950's diner and that's when my new career started.

Pulling up to the diner, Snake and I parked our jet black rental Camaro in a spot away from the building. Snake needed to smoke a cigarette, something he did compulsively. His oxygen was cigarettes. I also think he was bitching about the car standing out, which I later agreed was probably not the best choice if we wanted to blend in. Snake wasn't totally useless, but if I look back on it now I would have made him the fall guy.

We walked into the diner, always being aware of our surroundings, and we sat in a booth. Five, ten minutes go by and no Christmas. There is, however, an overweight white guy with big knotty dreadlocks sitting at the counter drinking a cup of coffee and sticking out like a sore thumb. He was also watching us. I figured he was her muscle, in case things went bad. She eventually showed up, giving us some story about soccer practice. I later learned that all weed connections run tardy no matter how much money is being transacted. It's something you have to get used to.

So we shoot the shit with Christmas. She dragged out the experience even longer and told us to get a hotel room so we could make this happen and we drove down the street and checked into a Marriott. Since we had never met her before, I was not able to get any product on credit, but we worked out a really good deal and negotiated around four pounds or something. We drove back home, purchased an internet ad on a site called WeedMaps for 1000 bucks a month, bought a burner cell phone (one that you can throw in the garbage) and we were in business. It was that simple. Our client base grew exponentially and consistently every month. When you do things that you love it is very easy to be successful.

The craziness of running rogue for years took its toll on my sanity, my girlfriend at the time, my family, and, somewhere deep down inside, told me to get out before it was too late. I'm glad I listened. I had already had a a special task force that was created between Henderson and Las Vegas visit my home. The farm that I had been working on was raided by paramilitary police officers and really the only way to use all the knowledge that I had acquired was to go legit. At the time, consulting in the cannabis industry was becoming big business, so I contacted a lobbyist friend and pretty much had a seamless transition from running a delivery and transportation service to consulting for an independently wealthy cannabis investor.

I completed multiple projects with this client, everything from warehouse purchasing, working on build outs with engineers and electricians to designing his brand packaging and labeling, getting compensated massively in the process, but working every month with absolutely no contract and or plans for the future. Once we separated, I was basically back to square one, except I no longer had Snake living with me. I no longer had a girlfriend living with me, either. My obsession with success above all else had pushed her away. At the time I thought everything was collapsing, but in reality the slate was just being wiped clean. It's impossible to see rock bottom when you are standing on it.

It's hard to see the good in situations when we are in the midst of chaos. Removing ourselves from the situation or figuring out a way to look at what is going on from a non conditioned perspective is always the best way to attack stressful situations.

Oddly enough, the first time I was introduced to the concept of yoga as being badass both physically and spiritually was when I was living in Vegas with Snake. It might have been around 2013 because the new Ford Explorer had just come out and that's what Eddie had rented and driven in from California. Eddie had just gotten out of prison and was on a road trip with his cousins enjoying his freedom. At the time my gray area business was thriving and things were just a little crazy in my life to say the least. Eddie stayed the weekend and left abruptly one night, a little more on that in a second.

You see Eddie wasn't actually my friend; he was my roommate's friend from home, NYC, and, like I said, he had just gotten out of prison. He was a big time gambler, ran big games at home, and he knew people that I knew, so we decided to party it up for the weekend. And it was too crazy. There were strip club blowjobs, massage parlor butthole lickings, and at the end of the weekend I was somehow missing a brick of hash. If you are making judgments about me, just remember I wasn't the one who just got out of prison. My butthole wasn't getting licked, I promise you that. Also the sad thing is that In New York, your best friend will point a gun at you and rob you for a bag of money. This guy wasn't even close to a friend. However, that weekend made for good stories.

Before you think we are already going off the deep end, I promise you we are talking about spirituality here. Over drinks at the world famous Palomino, the only full nude full bar in Las Vegas, Eddie told me why he did a bid, or, for you normal people, why he went to jail. The poor unfortunate guy got snitched on, go figure. And by who? You guessed it, by dirty cops, which at the time he wasn't aware of... allegedly.

Now how did this nice Spanish kid from uptown get involved in this mess you ask yourself? Eddie ran a poker club in the the city. I don't think I need to tell you which one, because there is only really one city that matters. Anyway, this happened to be the same club that A-Rod was arrested in, if you didn't know what town I was referring to.

As the story goes, one night Eddie was leaving the club to go make a drop and a van pulls up. He gets a bag put over his head, taken to the East River, and from then on is making payments to some guys every week. Or else guess what? They are going to rob his club. It's not until those guys get arrested and snitch on Eddie that it comes out they were dirty NYPD cops. Eddie didn't get arrested until the dirty cops snitched on him.

Yeah, so the first time I ever thought that yoga might be a cool thing was because all the money from the club, or most of it, was getting pushed through a yoga studio uptown in Harlem. "Yo Dawg, Hot Bitches." That's what Eddie would tell me every time we took a shot. Eddie is also the only one to this day that I have seen do handstands and warrior twos in a strip club.

The point is that even though Eddie was a scum bag, had total disregard for any other human besides himself and his daughter, he got it. There was an audacious sense of freedom to his personality, not just because he just got out of jail, but because he was a yogi, paid his dues to society, and, it's hard to believe from that story, but in some way he was reformed.

Whatever it was that jail, yoga, years of not seeing his daughter, had done to him In some way he got it. I could tell he had hit rock bottom before and what he got out of all the years of craziness was prison, the opportunity for nothing but self reflection. He left prison with more self enlightenment, more self awareness, and he understood that everything you have can be taken away in the blink of an eye. So yeah, that was the first time that yoga showed up on my radar, from a Spanish guy with tattoos ripping his shirt off in the strip club, doing yoga poses, and popping headstand for the strippers.

CHAPTER FOUR
Self Transcendence, Worshipping Yourself

"If your practice does not bring you joy, you are not practicing correctly."
Thich That Hanh

The path you are about to take is one of surrendering all that you currently hold onto regarding beliefs, identity, and preconceived notions about yourself and the world. It's about letting go of everything, and what will emerge is the true version of yourself. It is the process and realization of letting your ego, bad habits, and prior beliefs die in order to become new. It's about being present in every moment, never taking anything for granted, and leaving the earth a better place than you found it. It's about the desire to know the deepest truths of your own existence, however you choose to get there.

In order to accomplish the connection between mind, body, and soul, we will use vigorous exercise, meditation, educated approaches to nutrition, and drugs, if need be. The goal is to create the best version of ourselves and experience the most out of our short lives with every available tool that modern technology and the old world have provided to us.

We could make the argument or start the conversation that living in today's period of time could be the easiest it has ever been since the dawn of humanity. Never has it been more convenient to be a human. Since the creation of mankind, whether you believe it was Adam and Eve, some alien experiment, a simulation, or just the randomness of the universe that all living beings ended up on this rock, allegedly hurtling through space on this plain that we have invented called time, it's pretty conclusive that this is the peak of recorded humanity thus far.

As I present that idea to you I am sitting here typing this manuscript on my Ikea couch, my legs stretched out on my Ikea ottoman, typing this manuscript on a MacBook pro,

Netflix in background, not playing anything, but on, showing me previews on the South Korean television I picked up on cyber Monday. I'm not worrying about the plague, there aren't any Kings' wars I am being called off to go fight hand to hand in, and generally, even the insane can find a roof or some sort of shelter over their head in our country. Like I said, it's good to be a human these days.

I could also make the argument that the current time we are living in is the hardest it has ever been since we have never been more removed from nature and with that our true selves. At the core of humanity is the need to connect. To connect with others, to connect with nature, and to connect with ourselves. We have never been more disconnected to each other and from what that little voice inside of us is saying to us each day... We seem to forget that at the base of it all, we are just animals. Eat, sleep, shit, fuck. The basic programing of all living beings.

Somehow we still are part of nature, though. Most of us are living as ants in an ant farm. We wake up, technology addicted, subconsciously anticipating and building up anxiety, preparing for the sound of our digital alarm to go off each and every morning just so we can go to a job we hate. Sometimes, unexpectedly and for no reason at all, our alarm gets changed to a nuclear bomb alarm preventing us from ever really having any deep sleep again. Controlled by the machine.

We shower, well most of us, and get ready for the day. We walk into Starbucks immediately and almost involuntarily reaching for our phone, knowing that everyone is staring at us, the vain human that we are. Taking solace in the fact that if we pretend to check our emails we are invisible. A stranger says, "Hello," we pay them zero attention... scrolling or maybe even just staring at the nothingness in our hand. Paying it forward only when we are feeling guilty about something in our lives or when we think it can benefit us somehow.

40

We come home after a long day at the office of doing nothing, sitting on our asses, not having to kill anything, not having to walk for maybe two to three days before we eat, and we plop our decaying, sickly, GMO filled living carcass on the lazy boy, cracking open an energy drink, pulling up some app, ordering with our thumbs, never once saying a word, secretly complaining to ourselves in our head that it's not really delivery if they don't deliver to you on the couch. Paying with a fingerprint. It makes perfect sense why people are after enlightenment. I was stuck in that ant farm for over a decade.

There is no one formal organized text for what or how self enlightenment, self transcendence or, to sum it up, how self improvement is achieved or really what it is. We have all obviously heard of books like the Bible, the Torah, and the Koran, but this is an entirely different ballgame. As scholars we can all agree that if one chooses religion, its text can be used as a guide or set of principles in which one can, if they choose, live their life. What I am going to talk to you about is a little different. We are going to dive into the practice of self worship. The religion of you where there are no rules. And if you choose, over time that practice of self worship, self education will lead you to actually worshipping and believing in yourself.

If you are a religious person and think that this is just blasphemous, remember that you are created in his or her likeness. So in essence worshiping yourself is worshiping your god, but why limit yourself to just one god when they all have so much to offer?

If we are going to break it down in simple terms, self worship is figuring out and doing things that you love and that make you happy. It's about making yourself better. You are not going to be happy all the time. Being happy one hundred percent of the time is just unrealistic. If you were happy all of the time you would never be unhappy, thus never appreciating what true happiness really is.

You are going to include things in your life every day that make you a better person with the end result being growth. The key to this book, the key to really any type of success, is to be mindful in and of the present moment.

Before I go any further, I think it is important to address why we are discussing this topic. In recent months, I have been acutely aware of the use of the word enlightenment in popular culture. It has been showing up any my social feeds, I see the word in print ads and it's something that people have a very hard time grasping. If you do an internet search on the word enlightenment, let's say on the website Quora, a place where people can post questions about anything, there are tens of thousands of questions on the subject. People are obsessed with enlightenment and awareness. I think what is really going on is that people are looking for a spiritual realization, an awakening. People are looking for the ability to access a piece of their mind that is void of any religion, separate from any belief system, and open to mysteries of what being human is. They are just not categorizing it correctly. I believe you can find enlightenment through nutrition, exercise, and self exploration.

Enlightenment is not a real thing, it can't be had, it's not a cell phone. For it to become adaptable to popular culture and easier for the stupid people to swallow it up, enlightenment gets whittled down to #woke. Further removing us from the actual root word or goal of taking on such a difficult task. Just like there are conversations and debates on, for example, if Buddhism and Rastafarianism are religions or ways of life, enlightenment is just that... Whatever it means to you.

For what we are trying to learn and accomplish here, the word enlightenment with regards to hacking our body has to do with the goal of becoming mindful. Making being present in every moment the top priority of your life. Mindful of thoughts, mindful of time, mindful of space, mindful of where your food comes from and what you are putting into your body, mindful of everything.

At the heart and base of these practices is loving yourself and not feeling sorry for being selfish from time to time. You can't take care of others if you don't take care of yourself. Plain and simple.

To reach success in our endeavor there will be a bit of trial and error as everyone is different and we are creating our ideal vision of ourself. This does not happen overnight but we are not reinventing the wheel and have tools and examples from traditional religions, ways of life, and trains of thought that we can pull from.

All of us will start this journey thinking we kinda have an idea of where we think we should end up. I want to lose weight. I want to feel better about myself. I want to not be depressed, but at best this is wishful thinking for as we experience new things, old things, all things, the path in front of us will forever be changing. If I have learned anything from this journey, it is that nothing is set in stone.

CHAPTER FIVE
Take Back Control Of Your Life

"Refuse to live and die as another insignificant man." Tyrese

If you like being told what to do, asking permission to use the bathroom, and being told when you can feed yourself, that is fine. But life is about being your own person, your own boss, your own creator, your own god. There is nothing noble about being a caged dog, someone who is on a leash, who allows himself to be told when to piss, when to show up, and when to take a lunch. You should always be showing up. If you are taking a check and doing something that you don't believe in, you have lost your soul. I have been there.

What does being independent even mean? For me, for our purposes, it means being able to do whatever you want to do, when you want to do it, while always keeping intentions pure, not letting yourself get fucked over on the way. Hopefully, leaving society a little better when you kick the can… return to sender.

If you feel like your life sucks right now or that you are following a career path that doesn't keep you fulfilled, stop and think, why is that? Maybe you think you want a total restart. Well, you are right and you are wrong. You need to do more than just think about making a change. You NEED to do it!

The majority of humans come to this planet with one outcome: suffering an existence that is not fulfilling. They wake up every day knowing they are going to spend the rest of their conscious existence completing monotonous tasks that not only do little to improve society, but also won't help them feel better about themselves.

If you feel like a cog in the machine, it's because you are a cog in the machine and your true self is speaking to you. After I graduated from business school, the corporate world became my life. For more than 12 years, I woke up each day to a voice telling me that I was on the wrong path. Sometimes telling me to end it. It wasn't until I started doing literally whatever I wanted, never putting other people's timelines or wellbeing at risk, that the downward spiral reversed or at least seemed to slow down. The search for your true self is part of becoming your true self. It's a rough but necessary path that must be traveled and might never have a completion. It's your job to grit your teeth and carry on, no matter what.

You're gonna read this book and realize that your greatness has been inside of you the entire time. Not just since you started reading, but since birth. You may deny it, but most people - like you - have leadership in their genes. Don't believe it? That's because you are doing things that don't speak to your true self, that you are pissed off and have low self-esteem and question your value. I did this for over a decade, playing the corporate America game, not advancing my personal growth. I learned a lot about business in that decade, but even though I was relatively successful, I was never happy with my work. I never, ever fit in.

When you live and work in ways that don't speak to your true self, you are left unfulfilled at night, not excited to wake up in the morning. Life just plain sucks. You know that. I know that. And that's why a lot of us go and feed our demons on the weekend.

We all know what speaks to us in our lives, some of us are just more ready to go take it. By all means, if I wasn't meant to do what I am doing now and I just bit my tongue most of the time, I would still be sitting in an office, not doing much work, and getting paid relatively well for a job half done. I'd also be waking up every morning gasping for air Monday through Friday wanting to hang myself. I'd be spending my day doing busy work to fill the nine hours under the artificial lights planning my escape from captivity. For me it took multiple attempts and devastations of small fortunes to get back on the correct path. The information here includes what I have learned over the past five years to help me get back on the correct journey.

I don't know what the secret to life is, but I can tell you from my own experience that creating happiness, setting goals, and putting yourself in positions not only to succeed, but also to test yourself and possibly fail will help you figure it out. In a nutshell, DO THE WORK. Anything that we "fail" at is really just a lesson in an endeavor that did not speak to our true potential.

Just like the ant wakes up in the morning and does what it does, the beaver wakes up to build a dam, or the bee collects pollen to make honey, humans are meant to be working and doing what they are genetically programed to do. For me, it is to create and to teach. Only you know what your true self wants, where self enlightenment waits, but I can guarantee it's not the hustle and bustle of working for someone you don't even know.

The strategies I use and will lay out have led me out of the "depressed, funk downward spiral, waste of life, useless" periods in my life. And coincidentally, they are also the strategies, systems, and theories that allow me to keep a harmonious and positive energy in this universe. Waking up is no longer a chore.

CHAPTER SIX
Focus On The Present You

"Men do not attract that which they want, but that which they are."
James Allen

Many of our major struggles stem from the fact that we want to be good. We want to live with a purpose, help others, and lead by example. In reality, no one really gives a fuck about you.

In my own personal experience, I bent over backwards for people, for a cause. Multiple times, I placed the goals and aspirations of others well above my own. While there were successes, I also experienced setbacks on my career path. At times, my own ego took over, giving others too much information about myself, or over thinking things. I was the creator of my destruction. It was no one else's fault.

I have worked for hardcore narcissists, border line sociopathic CEO's, as well as the somewhat normal, independently wealthy entrepreneurs. Having learned the truth about business and life through these experiences, I have documented many self destructive patterns as well as patterns of success. This book is designed to give you a blueprint, some suggestions, anecdotes, and maybe some stories about how I got to where I am today. If you are trying to find yourself or improve your life, this book, hopefully, will be more than just a fun read. Patterns are everywhere around us and when we decide to take notice of them or, even better, document them, real learning can begin. That's where the journey starts.

When I was younger I was tested for learning disabilities. And because of that for a long time I believed that that something was wrong with me. I always knew then and obviously know now that's not true. What is true is that if a subject, topic, or conversation is not interesting to me, I have almost no ability to focus on it. The opposite is true for subjects that I love. I am easily able to dive into them and master them with relative ease. This is my super power.

My specific learning disability had to do with rote memorization, which is basically the ability to recall numbers, names, and shit like that at the drop of the hat. I had to learn early on that there were other ways to process information. Contextual learning is exactly what it sounds like: doing the activity and learning by trial and error. I have also learned that if we go through life telling ourselves one thing, that idea will become part of our life.

So from personal experience and observations of every human in my life, I concluded that the root of all of our problems stems from self esteem. But is self esteem even a real thing? I tend to say no as it is primarily based not off of what we think of ourselves, but what we think that others think of us, meaning that our reality is being shaped by what most likely doesn't even exist. And if it does who cares? As the Chinese philosopher Lao-Tzu stated, "If you are depressed you are living in the past. If you are anxious, you are living in the future. If you are at peace you are living in the present." This book is about living and focusing on the present.

Take Inventory and Answer Some Questions

"Thoughts become things." Kai Greene

Look at your home or apartment, look at your car, look at your pets. Everything that you own or associate yourself with is a direct reflection of you. A direct reflection of your thoughts and a direct reflection of what is going on inside your head. When I was close to 300 pounds, with a messy apartment, dirty car, and a pit bull the size of a wild hog, it was a clear indication that something was destroying me from the inside. It was also manifesting itself on the outside with my appearance.

48

Look at your dog. Your dog doesn't have an opinion of its self worth. It just is. It knows the basic concept of right and wrong (thanks to you) and has no inclination of "I'm awesome," or "I'm a shitty dog," or "man, am I going to get that promotion?" In fact, a clear argument can be made that your pet is ONLY living in the present. I'm going to encourage you to think like the animals because, after all, that is what we are, animals.

Be like the dog and think about what is happening to you right now and only right now. A dog does not care what others think of it. A dog is just existing. Dogs have clearly evolved to only exist in the present. A dog's only intention is pleasing its master. Yet, I can unequivocally guarantee that your dog is not sitting on the couch right now creating anxiety about how it is going to please you when you get home.

Our goal is to embrace our animalistic state and not let the ideas, the jealousy, and personification of what others think we should do affect us. The goals and aspirations of what others have for you will never serve you. What we are aiming to create is a life that serves our purpose.

Now is your chance to reclaim your power. Live in your paradox and create your life. If it wasn't for the first path that you took, the path that others gave you, you would not have come to this crossroad. Seeing that the path that we embraced was not for us, we are at a different place and time in our life. A place of rebirth and recreation. This book is about recreating the new you.

Begin by completing these short exercises.

Identify The 4 Emotions That will Change Your Life:
1. **Disgust:** "I've had it! Enough is Enough."
2. **Decision:** "I am going to do everything in my power, maybe be a little more uncomfortable at times, but I am going to change my life for the better."
3. **Desire:** How bad do you want it? What is the spark for you desire? Is it a conversation you need to have? Welcome all experience as you never know what will turn it on. I have found that sometimes changing your life is as easy as asking for it.
4. **Resolve:** I will. Stake you existence on your purpose + DO OR DIE. LEARN, GROW, CHANGE, BECOME.

FOUR Questions To Ask Yourself Right Now:
1. What am I good at?
2. What am I marginal at?
3. What do I suck at?
4. What vision of my life do I have?

Our goal in life should be to identify our weaknesses, figure out the boundaries of our skill levels and blast right through them. Being human is about constant evolution. This book is designed to give you a blueprint for your physical and spiritual success.

CHAPTER SEVEN
Why Are Experts Important?

"Learn of the skillful; he who teaches himself, has a fool for a master."
Benjamin Franklin

I was that fool until I started hiring experts to help me get to the next level.

Alright. So you woke up. Or at least you are beginning to. Turned on to the thought that you have something greater to do, more to add to this earth than what you are currently contributing. I don't know what that is and you might not either, but I want you to be able to tell me at some point what that is. Better yet, I want you to show me and lead by example. If you are born with greatness you know it, you feel it, people follow you whether you want them to or not. Believe me that is the story of my life.

I am stronger today because of the obstacles I have encountered in the past. I'm going to share these details so you can better understand my own transformation and how I have come to be able to help others. I've done the hard work. Maybe you'll see some of yourself in what I'm telling you. In any case, you can benefit from my experience and insight.

My path began as far back as kindergarten when I got pulled out of class by Ms. Myers. "Joe, do you want to be the class clown all your life? You're not paying attention and you do whatever you want and, in turn, all the other kids are losing their attention and copying you. Do you want to be the class clown?"

I think we were coloring or something and that shit just didn't appeal to me. At home I was cooking Italian meals from scratch and building telephones with my dad. Coloring at the time was beneath. Even as a small kid the teacher's comment didn't make sense to me. Class clown? I remember having the same conversation with the head of the lower school and I wondered why I got in trouble for doing whatever I wanted. Was it my fault that all the turds in the class were following me and not the teacher?

Another example: in 6th grade I was in a summer camp. I was physically pulled out of a men's locker room by the head of the camp. In the 1990's juice was legal and the head of the camp was a guy named Rob who was a fucking monster. I was dragged out like a rag doll to the same conversation. "Joe, you realize all these kids do whatever you do and when you just do your thing that affects the other kids and they start to misbehave." I remember telling Rob that I didn't want to be a leader and I made up an excuse as to why I didn't want to participate in the activities at hand. I didn't think I should be held responsible for other kids following my lead.

I was never a brat. But as a kid I would always give thought to what I was told and most of the time I would do the opposite. I just never believed in being a sheep, in doing things that I really didn't want to do and that, according to society, was my problem. I was an exceptional swimmer growing up even though I was a fat kid. But in any reality I could imagine, death was a better alternative to wearing a Speedo and joining a swim team. I eventually negotiated myself onto the tennis team and that became one of the highlights of my life, playing tennis, traveling and competing above my age group. Tennis is not a team sport and it's not surprising that everything I have excelled at has been a one man show.

Why Blood, Sweat, and Years?

"You have to be willing to suffer." James Allen

Why *Blood, Sweat, and Years?* Well, for one I think it's catchy, but at the end of the day that is what your journey is going to take. It's going to take hard work. Blood signifies our suffering, sweat, the hard work that needs to get done to get where we want to go and years representing the life long process and lifestyle we are committing to. Always keeping in mind that we only have a certain amount of time on this earth and no clue what the expiration date is.

I went to three high schools, the first one being in NYC where I eventually got arrested for smoking a joint. This happened in the late 1990s. I was probably 15 and on an early fall night was hanging out in a park with about 30 other teens. Four of us were pinpointed as the center of the group. (Mistaken identity again?) After I was off of probation, the case now expunged, my parents immediately had me sent to Utah to a place called RedCliff Ascent. RedCliff was the first taste I had of being human, being a man, and seeing what true humanity is really like. Seeing what people are like when they are desperate and broken down. Living in the desert taught me everything I needed to know about survival and the true soul of men.

To fully understand the experience I will set your plate:

As soon as you get off of probation and are allowed to leave the state your parents hire professional kidnappers. I was lucky to have a nice mixed couple of kidnappers, meaning a 6'8 black dude and a 6'5 white guy.

I was introduced to them when my door was slammed open and I was wakened from a dead sleep. I had gotten off of probation the day before and my "boys" had smoked me out. I was still had a weed hangover. I don't remember the time, but it was for sure early. So the door busts open, two goons come in the room, my mom is sobbing and my dad is trying to console her. (I'm confused, I'm outnumbered with nowhere to go. Sill under my covers.) I know I fucked up, but shit I just got off probation. I thought I had done my time. Also why are my parents crying? They are the ones who let these guys into the house.

So the kidnappers introduce themselves and proceed to go in my closet, hand me a pair of jeans, a white t-shirt, and my Timberlands. I ask to use the bathroom and they go into the bathroom, opening the windows, looking under the toilet seats, removing any bathrobe belts, and tell me to pee with the door open. I asked them why they needed to do that and they responded, "Sometimes you kids have a knife in there or something." I'm thinking to myself, "What the fuck? I got arrested for a joint not assault and battery. This is nuts."

As soon as we get into the car the comments start coming. "Oh shit man, your parents are rich, why didn't they let us sleep in the house?" (I'm adopted, my parents, came from nothing, and this has been the "quintessential" put down I have heard all my life.) I responded, "Fuck you man." The kidnappers flew me to Vegas, a place I now live in, a place I tried to run, and then eventually to Utah where, for the next 92 days, I learned what it was to be human. I learned what it was to fend for yourself spending many nights alone in the desert on what was called solo. Our solos were supposed to last 24 hours, but sometimes the sun would rise and fall two or three times before anyone came out to check on us. I learned very quickly what it was like to be alone and fend for yourself. I have learned to be alone and this is something that is hard for most people to even fathom enjoying.

RedCliff was a very unpleasant experience at first. I was arrested once for smoking a joint and spent less than a night in a holding cell, however, I never have and don't plan on going to prison. That is just general good advice for anyone. I imagine that prison is somewhat similar as far as structure to that of a wilderness program. Essentially you have no identity and you are just a number.

The process starts with the goons dropping you off handing you over to the leader of the program. In my case he went by Black Bear. They then proceed to take you into the basement of a cabin/office building and begin to process you.

54

The processing involves you stripping naked, the whole nine yards, you spread your buttcheeks, you cough, they check your insoles, you lift up your nuts, all that shit. The whole experience, the whole business is about stripping away your ego. Anyway I sleep butt naked. You want me to pull up my dick, check under my balls, and fart on you, no problem.

So you go through that rigamarole and they give you your supplies, two water bottles, some food that needs to be hydrated, a pound of rice, a pound of lentils, and chicken bouillon. You get a metal cup, a wool blanket, a sleeping bag, a tarp and some shoe string. "Alright guys where is the backpack I put this in?" "No, no, you see you have to earn your backpack here." You tie your pack up in your tarp with the shoe string, and you use seatbelt straps for shoulder harnesses.

You're sent to base camp, where you are called a pollywog, meaning you are new to this world and have no legs to swim, like a frog. Base camp is a bitch. you are either there with new people, people who have gotten injured, or people who have been there for a while for some reason or another and or are getting transferred elsewhere. You have also just essentially been kidnapped, been stripped naked, and have been blindfolded and driven to the middle of the desert. Needless to say the whole situation is a little stressful and for sure very confusing.

Base camp is far, or it could not be far. I still don't know. After you are butt searched you are blindfolded and put into a shit box suburban and driven to your camp. Most likely you are probably driven around in circles, but it feels like they drive you for about an hour. The program's headquarters is about an hour from two major wilderness areas. Then halfway through the ride they say, "Ok you can look." The moment that you open your eyes and are adjusting to the light, they re-blindfold you, further trying to break you down.

So we get to base camp. I'm a pollywog, a city boy, and I don't fuck with any of this shit. Immediately this Spanish kid comes up to me, asking to trade his rice for my raisins. At this time in my life I was not a fan of rice at all, but I didn't want any trouble. I also didn't want to seem like a bitch, AT ALL. The trade sounded fair, but you can't hustle the hustlers and being from New York I made him throw in a roll of toilet paper on the deal.

We eventually ended up in the same group and named it the Lone Wolves. Our group was the savages out of all the groups. We were known to hike 10-12 miles a day like soldiers and spend days in the middle of nowhere where we would eat our rations, but also hunt with figure four traps, eating rats and birds we had killed with rocks, also make netting for rivers that we had found where we would catch crawdads. It was some primal shit. The only things missing were spears and Wooly Mammoths. To this day I still maintain the savage. Most people never get to experience this part of being human. You will after this book.

When I got to RedCliff I was dead last on all hikes, lazy, and entitled. The average kidnappee is there for 30 days. I was there for 91 or 92 I can't remember. From a little fat kid who started off at the back of the march I ended up the group leader rather quickly, getting access to maps, getting close enough to counselors to steal toothpaste and tobacco, and finding that raw power from the ancestors. I saw a lot of people quit there. I saw a lot of people succumb to being human. Most of the people in my group are now dead as well. Most of my closest friends coincidentally are dead, too. If you're here you've probably been around the block, too.

Everyone should be sent or at least spend some time in the desert. In today's society we are getting further and further away from the wild. Do some serious introspection away from technology. Spending time in nature will remind you of what your purpose truly is. If you can't travel to a desert, the woods should do it for you, but I highly recommend spending some time alone away from the maddening crowds of society.

"If you can't fly, then run, if you can't walk run, then walk, if you can't walk, then crawl, but by all means keep moving." Martin Luther King Jr.

I graduated from RedCliff, being given a spirit name of Smiling Bull Charging, meaning one who goes after everything full force and full steam with a smile on his face. Well Smiling Bull thought he was charging back to New York City and instead of the original deal, was sent to a place called Hyde School.

Marketing is a crazy thing. Hyde, which is in Connecticut and no longer exists, was branded and marketed as a character education school. However, what it should have been called was Guantanamo Bay Boarding School. Most of the tactics they employed on us would no longer be acceptable in today's marshmallow society.

I am forever thankful for torture school because it is what made me the man I am today. I have literally never faced mental or physical pain as serious as the ones that I faced day in and day out in Connecticut. No challenge, no matter how great in my life after high school, has been even 10% of the craziness, the ego dissolution, and literal torture of mind and body that I experienced in Connecticut. Hyde is probably why I never killed myself when the going got tough. I had faced what I would call real pain.That place was tough. I even got kicked out of there.

I can remember one night when there was a theft on the wing of my dorm. The solution was to pack all 28 members of that wing into one room, having everyone bring their alarm clocks into the room and have us sit on the floor with all the alarms blaring until someone ratted someone else out. They were only interrogating half of the real suspects since two wings were connected through a bathroom. If you had a problem with their methods they threatened us with being put out in the snow in our underwear and made to stand outside the window of the room with the alarm clocks. That's what I chose. I'm dumb, but in my experience, my preference is being tortured in solitude rather than in a group setting.

A little background on the school's philosophy:

At the heart of the school is an ideology which makes sense - character, integrity, brother's keeper, all that jazz. It's great in theory, however this school was run by a crazy old man and his family. The premise was that your parents sent you to a place that looked like a boarding school, however you are with about 300 to 400 other "troubled teens" in this facade of a boarding school.

I never went to a traditional boarding school. I imagine if you get in trouble in boarding school you get detention. At Hyde you would go into a program called 2-4, meaning 24, meaning 24 hours a day. Think of a chain gang. Your job is to wake up at 5 a.m. and do a torture workout (bootcamp) called a 5:30, then instead of doing your scholastic duties, you are in the field, or the woods, or on the plain, cutting trees, digging holes, cleaning toilets, "building character." If the group is acting up, you would have more workouts in the field, sometimes never stopping until everyone is puking. Coincidentally, this is the form of exercise I now teach at a high level. Except instead of torture I use positivity to build people up by putting thought into the choreography of my classes. It's not just bear crawls and mountain climbers. Our workouts were led by an ex-navy guy who got off on trying to break us down. I mean the guy would even suit up in football pads during season and go full force against the JV guys. A real winner of a human.

I personally had multiple incidences where I would end up spending weeks on this duty because the harder you come at me the harder I go. Sometimes even getting in trouble on 2-4, think about that. This is the mentality I want you to have. Never give up on yourself, especially when the going gets tough. Always be yourself. Always keep to your vision. Especially when others are being malicious towards your success. Remember, no one really gives a fuck about you. It's your job to do just that. GIVE A FUCK.

Needless to say I got in trouble a lot. I smoked pot, I had sex with girls, I didn't obey lights out, pretty much the standard 16 year old stuff. This meant I would spend weeks at a time on 2-4. After a while school became 2-4, not classes. I enjoy working out and I like working hard so the risk-reward ratio was clear. If I hook up with chicks, or get high, or anything that was against the rules, I got in trouble. Meaning, I got to work out and do manual labor all day, plus not go to school. It wasn't an ideal situation, but I had to adapt during those weeks.

Eventually when they figured out that 2-4 didn't work I got sent to a place called the Black Wilderness Preserve which was a 10-day experience in "hell." However, my time in Utah was a lazy Sunday compared to their version of "HELL." I had the privilege of visiting the Black Wilderness Preserve twice, never once telling them that I loved snowshoeing. At some points in your life when the going gets really tough, when your body is in pain and you feel like giving up, you have to realize that the worst thing that can happen is death, and that you just have to keep pushing through that fear. If you do die everything that you think is a problem in right now, just isn't.

What do I want you to take away from my experience? That's on you to decide. Perhaps it means not being so hard on yourself if you don't conform to society's idea of what your life should be like. Maybe to take to heart that saying, "no pain, no gain." Maybe you always choose the road less traveled for some reason. There's no right or wrong way to forge your path, even though most people will NOT understand what you are up to. It's extremely important to be calculated in everything you do no matter how crazy it might seem to the outside world. You always have to be aware of the end game. If you look at the top artists, leaders, and businessmen in the world, one thing they all have in common is strength, courage, and a determination to keep going and be the best. It's a constant battle not only for gains, but against losses.

CHAPTER EIGHT
Finding Your Passion

"I owe my success to having listened respectfully to the very best advice, and then going away and doing the exact opposite." G. K. Chesterton

When I was a kid I wanted to do whatever I wanted and without being disciplined. Oddly enough, what I have learned, is that the key to being able to do whatever you want, most of the time, means having an extreme amount of discipline all of the time. I am now a firm believer in schedules and have even left meetings, doctor's appointments, whatever, in order to keep my day productive, to keep in line with how I envision my life as a productive human being. When there is free time, which I control, I schedule meetings with myself where I do work. Always have discipline… always have freedom. Always keep yourself busy with new projects or hobbies.

After graduating from college in 2006, I worked in corporate America. In 2017, I had a full time, 50-hour a week shitty corporate job with a 100 year-old company, with all the benefits and the perks of a soda machine, health insurance, and a one-hour unpaid lunch. However, this was the year I started instructing fitness and everything changed. I taught boot camps and pilates classes on my two days off. I did a total of four classes a week, every week, on top of the job for the entire year. 1.5 jobs is not a crazy feat, but during that time I started to create a yoga clothing line for men because I couldn't find any dope gear to wear to classes. It wasn't that I wanted to start a yoga clothing company, it was that I needed pants to wear to class that weren't just black. In that December, I started making orders for samples and I quit teaching. I became obsessed. Be obsessed with your passions. Be obsessed with your success. If you can't be obsessed with your own shit, you are wasting your time. If you fail and you absolutely know that you have given it your all, it just wasn't meant to be.

Teaching group fitness was a way for me to get a foot in the door and if it wasn't for teaching no one would be reading this because HeatSeekerYogi wouldn't exist. Lesson: Always be manifesting visions of your ideal future, but have no attachment to it. Constantly thinking about the future builds anxiety and tension in the body. Also, it is good to have an idea of where you want to end up, but most likely you will be close, but not on the money. Don't be attached to the end goal either. Just add value.

At the time that HeatSeekerYogi was brewing I had a need to "feel alive" (for lack of a better term), so I got a little off track and I started running obstacle course races. I hired the best bodybuilding and nutrition coaches, read as much as I could, and somewhere along the line got the obstacle course racing bug big time. I did a few events and did fairly well, competing in the non competitive field in all events, thinking I was awesome.

Somewhere along the line my dream of helping people switched to obstacle course racing, shifting me vastly off course. However, it taught me a valuable lesson in goal setting. Mainly… Don't stray from the plan.

I truly enjoy obstacle course racing, but I have no business running with the best in the world. I competed in an Elite event and from the second the gun went off it was a nightmare.

Like a stampede of buffalos, we were out the gate. I am truly honest with my capabilities and for the first 20 yards I'm like Flash Gordon, the fastest human in the world. However, as I am gassing out on my sprint, amidst the herd of jurassic park dinosaurs, the sea of humans started to split. Out of nowhere I saw a cameraman and his assistant on their knees directly in front of me as if the assistant was using the camera man as a shield in the movie "300." Out of 278 people, some chose left, some chose right, I chose straight and leveled the camera man, completely devastating him and causing me to roll another 10 or 15 feet, creating a pile up and earning me one of the most intense headaches I have ever had. I was out for the count after that.

To save face, my body dumped all of my adrenaline out and I got up, but I was clearly done for the race. Out of 278 people I came in 272, or 271. If we are putting all the cards on the table, I only saw one guy behind me so I figure a few dudes didn't show up and maybe one guy broke his leg in that pile up. I don't know.

The point of that rant is that the universe is going to hit us sometimes with a big ass sledgehammer. You're on point. You make a plan and in my case it said to me, "Joe, go ahead and try this this out. You have been working on your business for almost two years, writing is going well, now you want to go do some mud running and change the entire direction of your plan? Ok? But is that what you really want to do?" The answer was no. After the race I decided to still sell to racers, but primarily focus on yoga, teaching, and the lifestyle aspect of my business.

There is nothing wrong with veering off the path as long as we realize that sticking to the original plan is always the best idea and that any type of detour is really just a lesson into what we do want, but don't need. I need to be teaching and creating dope gear. I don't need to be traveling around running races at this point in my life. It is important to make a goal and stick with it. I ran elite. I ran like shit. It's all good.

Through racing I came back to yoga and, more importantly, teaching. Through yoga I went on a retreat to Hawaii. Because of Hawaii I was able to muster up the courage to quit working in my cubicle. I was able to let go of being what most people consider "safe."

These days I now have the pleasure of choosing to wake up at 6:30 or 7 a.m. every day, just like I did when I was working for the man. However, my day is now mine. I go get coffee whenever the fuck I want. I get to take one to two classes a day if I choose or go to the gym. The laptop lifestyle, running most if not all of my business out of my home, storing all my products at the amazon warehouse. And I get off on see-ing lifestyle clients create their vision for their dreams. It's selfish, but helping others achieve their goals gets me off.

Being happy is a goal; it is not something you can be 100% of the time. In order to create these moment of "happiness" we have to be constantly challenging ourselves and putting our-selves in places to not only succeed, but to learn valuable lessons in failure at the same time. Maybe that is why I chose obstacle racing for that short period of time. I don't know. Life will usually always give us an opportunity for the test when things become monotonous or like the movie "Groundhog Day." It's up to us to take advantage of those events. If we are constantly on the pursuit of self betterment, the challenges will come to us.

Setting Expectations

"People who succeed have momentum. The more they succeed, the more they want to succeed, and the more they find a way to succeed. Similarly, when someone is failing, the tendency is to get on a downward spiral that can even become a self-fulfilling prophecy." Tony Robbins

So you got a little bent out of shape… The hot chick doesn't want to go on a date with you. Or maybe you really wanted that promotion at the "job" that you think you love and you got passed over by someone who plays the game better than you. Maybe you work at a used car dealership and you have a dad bod and drink too much beer at night.

Wait… Or better yet, you have it all figured out, man. You have a mortgage on a dope condo, a shitty entry level Ger-man car, a couple pieces of designer Italian nonsense, and a really hot young thang living with you. Maybe, you even get a little crazy and do some blow on the weekends. I know, I did.

You're cool man. I know I was. Now ask yourself, are you fulfilled? Chances are if you are reading this you're not. Or, you could be just curious about what I have to say.

At this moment in time your lifestyle and image are probably everything to you. And it's so basic and cliché, but in the blink of an eye or the proverbial drop of a hat, one misjudgment in life and the entire world that you have created can fall apart. Or you just let it go to shit. That's what I did.

If that has happened to you or you fear you are in a downward spiral, don't worry. The version of the life you are living right now is not in harmony with who you really are. That's why shit isn't working.

The frequency of who you are and the frequency of your current state of life are not in alignment. The harder you push to get into alignment the deeper and more out of control your spiral will feel. Been there, done that, hated it…..

Let yourself hit the bottom, whatever that means to you and I promise you two things. If we look at the bottom of any staircase or elevator there is usually an exit door (which I don't recommend anyone take, so let's get that out of the way), but there is also a bottom floor. Use the floor as a new foundation to build… well, whatever the hell version of you you want. It's that simple.

The idea of a *Blood, Sweat, and Years* is to become the best version of yourself, coincidentally bringing the levels of other's true selves up in the process, sometimes without them even knowing. You are a natural born leader who intoxicates the people around you. People instinctively follow you. Once we have hit bottom we have the opportunity to reevaluate everything in our lives and create whatever version of ourselves that we want. That is the beauty of restarting.

These days, it's cool to say you don't have any expectations. It's a protective device. If you expect something and it doesn't happen, you won't be let down, but that is a fucking cop out. I insist that you have the highest expectations, not only for yourself, but for others as well. For everyone that you surround yourself with. However, we should also be realistic and be prepared for let downs if they do come, acting rational and with peace of mind for those inevitable events when things don't always go our way. Sri Chinmoy was once quoted as saying, "Peace begins, when expectations end." I implore you to integrate that into your life.

You have been talking to this beautiful woman, maybe she is even your "soul mate." You have taken it slow and there is a huge sexual tension built up between the two of you. You finally get the nerves or balls to ask her out. She agrees to this weekend, and you are psyched. You make it casual, a cool brewery pizzeria, something you have talked about before and just to be the good guy, you confirm the night before as it has been a few days since you last saw each other and spoke. The weekend comes. You bought a fresh pair of Levis, cut your hair, trimmed your bush, and 32 minutes before you are supposed to meet, as you are trimming that bush you hear, ding ding. It's your text message. Paying no mind you finish your business. You dry off, look at the phone, and she has canceled.

Now of course the expectation was that you were going to have a nice evening out with a friend and even possibly get laid. However, the universe had something else in store. In the story above everything was planned to the minute. You made plans, you confirmed, you set the expectation of a beautiful evening. Maybe that was too much? Maybe you shouldn't have confirmed. Maybe the restaurant was the wrong place. What did you do wrong? The answer is nothing.

The only mistake here was placing the happiness of your evening on someone else's shoulders. It is completely reasonable to have EXPECTED a great evening to turn out. You even planned for it That is where it should end. You did everything you could to create a great night. The only problem was expecting it to go off without a hitch.

That story above was obviously a personal anecdote to help conceptualize the idea, but did I get angry at my canceled date? Absolutely not. What did I do? I took myself out and had an amazing time by myself. For it's only with yourself that you can drop your guard and have zero expectations.

Throughout the pages of this book I am going to give you examples from my own life, but they may not all relate to yours. The idea is to understand that everyone struggles. Everyone has self esteem issues, weight loss issues, or question their existence at some point in their short time as a spec of dust in this universe. Our goal is to build a foundation that is higher than rock bottom for us to build upon.

When I was growing up and attacking a problem or a project, my dad would always say the same thing to me. And to this day I hear his voice ringing in the back of my head whenever I approach a project, "Joe, keep it simple." So that is what we are going to do. *Blood Sweat and Years* is about taking all the information that seems far out there and boiling it down into a simple recipe for you to create personal success, whatever success is to you - mental, physical, spiritual or all three.

I started my journey thinking I knew where I wanted to go. "I want to lose a little weight. I want to feel better. I want to fit into that whatever for that whatever." And as we see changes, as we become better versions of ourselves, our natural and totally healthy narcissistic human side comes out and it automatically translates the changes happening in our brain and body into our daily lives. My fat loss journey became one of a spiritual endeavor. Small changes are going to add up to mas-

67

sive links of success in a chain that essentially could go on forever. Our goal is not only to get rid of some of our bad habits, but to gain positive ones as well.

CHAPTER NINE
To Change Your Mind, Start with Your Body

"The successful warrior is the average man, with laser-like focus." Bruce Lee

If you are having trouble healing your mind then there is only one way to access that pain and it is directly through the body. The same works in reverse for the body. There are a couple ways you can go about things when it comes to completely recompositioning your body, your mind, and changing your life. The first step is that you have to want to make the change. Then you have two options. You can take the super fast and unhealthy unsustainable approach and have short-lived success. I've been there, and there was no longevity or enlightenment. Or you can take an educated approach and be in tune with your body, learn to listen to your body, and learn to know what it needs throughout the day.

I'll start off by saying something very cliché and even though it's not 100% true, it's as true as the times we live in. "I TRIED EVERY DIET." Atkins, Paleo, the all steak diet, the all eggs diet, the Mediterranean diet, the ketogenic diet, I even went as far as going vegetarian for six months when I was dating a super hot 20-something year-old vegan. No one hates "squishing" tofu more than I do. And guess what? All of those diets worked - for a time. And according to a UCLA study that followed dieters for at least two years, "83 percent gained back more weight than they had lost during those years… One study found that 50 percent of dieters weighed more than 11 pounds over their starting weight five years after the diet…" Their research concluded that, "People on diets typically lose five to ten percent of their starting weight in the first six months… However, at least one-third to two-thirds of people on diets regain more weight than they lost within four or five years, and the true number may well be significantly higher." [1]

So why is that? Why is the plan laid out in this book different? You will learn soon my friend, I promise.

The typical person usually goes into a diet or a workout routine with high ambitions. Once we achieve our goal, statistically we tend to lighten up a bit, get a little less hardcore and think, "Oh, ok I've lost 20 pounds. I'm looking good," eventually, maybe not going back to our old habits, but letting things slip here and there. Having an extra cheese burger, binging more than recommended, becoming a fatter lazier slob than we were before. All because the goal was reached, but we didn't have a plan or routine in place to maintain it. As the builders of the Tappan Zee Bridge built in 1952 found out, it's easy to build a bridge, it's a little harder to build it to maintain the test of time. So we want to design a plan of action that is going to have lasting results. We want to over engineer our body. Think of the Brooklyn Bridge in this analogy. Built in 1883 and probably going to end up as a world wonder hundreds of years from now long after we are dead.

You have probably been down this road before. We don't need to harp on the past. It technically doesn't exist. The past is just a mixture of chemicals and electromagnetic activity releasing and firing in our brain. In fact, please forget everything you know about "dieting" because this isn't a diet. What I am trying to get across is lifestyle, a choice, a plan and way of being in these confusing times. You have to be willing to put in the initial work and you have to be wiling to experiment on yourself. With that work, I guarantee you the side effects of your new lifestyle will be better health, a better physique, more mental clarity, and pretty much anything else

---

[1] Wolpert, Stuart. "Dieting does not work, UCLA researchers report." UCLA Newsroom. http://newsroom.ucla.edu/releases/Dieting-Does-Not-Work-UCLA-Researchers-7832. (7/5/2018)

that you want in life. It's all up to you. There is no magic pill. You also didn't buy snake oil. You just have to put in the work.

I have many experiences that I want to share with you and techniques I want you to know. With that said this is not a textbook, but I do have a fascination with nutrition, chemistry, and changing the body and mind. Everything that you will read I practice or have practiced at some point in my transformation journey. You can read the book, follow it to a T, or you can implement certain parts of it into your life. That's up to you.

Making The Commitment

"Exercise to stimulate not to annihilate. The world wasn't built in a day, and neither were we. Set small goals and build upon them." Lee Haney 8X Mr. Olympia

That quote can be applied to many aspects of our life. On my death bed I will ask myself this: "Did I leave the world better than I found it? Did we create something for the greater good?" It only matters to me that you want to get into the best physical and mental shape of your life. The two are one and the same. I am going to give you the tools you will need. Your dream body, your dream mindset, whatever your vision is. I'm going to figure it out for you. However, you are going to need to do all the hard work. Pablo Picasso was quoted as saying, "The meaning of life is to find your gift. The purpose of life is to give it away." Well, here it is.

My weight loss goal required me to not end up looking like a deflated garbage bag. I wanted to look like I fucking worked out. And as I continually make improvements, I have found that there really is no limit to functionality. If you apply the proper stresses to your body, it will only get as big and as muscular as needed. The human body is a miracle adaptation machine and responds directly to the stresses we are applying.

71

If you ask your body to do something multiple times, for example, lift a rock, it will through time adapt and grow to lift that rock. That's just how it works.

The program in here is pretty simple. The basis is yoga, bodybuilding, a solid nutritional foundation, and a little cardio when we see ourself getting fluffy (**FAT**). Part of our program stretches the muscles, contorting them in ways you have never imagined. Another packs on pure mass. And at the basis, nutrition which takes extreme mental discipline. All disciplines requiring the "connection" between the mind and muscles, all the disciplines being just that disciplines. What we lack at this point, our starting point, is discipline.

My goal physically is to obtain as much functional muscle as possible. After losing over 100 pounds I believe anyone can get healthy mentally and physically and keep it that way. They just have to be in it to win it. You just can't just make and use your current excuses to avoid pain.

On the quest for our best selves, we should be learning things about our bodies every day. I strongly suggest that you keep a journal of your progress and failures so you can learn from them. Even write how you feel mentally when waking up in the morning. In this day an age we should be collecting and using as much data as we can to reach our personal goals.

 All of the methods in this book are designed to work without the use of supplements or drugs. However, there is no question that drugs work. Consistency is the main component of the program. Without consistency we will never be successful in this transformation.

I ask you to have an open mind as I did when experimenting on myself. The information here is designed to help you and to provide you with methods that not only work, but make sense. I'm living proof that you can literally look like whatever you can imagine.

The whole point of being in the gym, fitness studio, this whole shit is to motivate each other. So however you choose to reach your goals just remember everyone is in it for the same reason, to be better than they were yesterday. The gym, the yoga studio, these places should be destinations where everyone can go and work on themselves. And more importantly be themselves.

The *Blood, Sweat, and Years* lifestyle focuses on listening to our bodies, learning what they are telling us, and giving our bodies the food, supplements, exercise, and mental stimulation needed to achieve peak performance living on a daily basis. This is just one way to be successful, but it's the way I, and the people I coach, are successful. Each and everyone's body is different and everyone will have to modify this program to meet their own personal needs. Or you can hire me and I'll set it up for you.

CHAPTER TEN
Keys to Success

"I think if you exercise, your state of mind - my state of mind - is usually more at ease, ready for more mental challenges. Once I get the physical stuff out of the way it always seems like I have more calmness and better self-esteem." Stone Gossard

Lose 14 pounds in seven days. Get big muscles in eight minutes or less a day with this widget you bought after seeing a TV commercial. Sign on for the non diet diet. Order your coffee on your app and pick it up in store. Read the Cliff-Notes. Watch the movie version of the book. This is the society we live in today. And all of those quick fixes appeal to the lazy, childish, gullible baby that we have inside of us.

I have often been criticized that my methods at times can be too simple, but weight loss and mental exploration is not rocket science. They are lifestyle choices. Here are the four platforms that we must adhere to in order to be successful.

Time: Nothing is going to work overnight I tell all my clients. If it took you 30 years to get fat, do you realistically believe that it will take three months to lose all your weight? I can tell you that getting fat is a full-time job. It's a lifestyle. The same goes with being depressed. That is why you have to make the decision to get in shape and mold your life around your goals. Mold you life around the vision you have for your future.

Consistency: This is the biggest one for me. I harp on this a lot. I tried most of the fad diets and when the diet was over, so was my progress. Our goal, our philosophy is to build rituals which we will adhere to in our daily lives. We want these rituals and good habits to become involuntary, like blinking. We want the good nutritional decisions to be the first thought that comes to our mind when we are hungry. And although we cannot change the neuro-pathways in our brain, we can create new ones with time. We want to create a new highway of positive thinking for those signals in our brain. The only way to do that is through repetition, believing that we can, and staying consistent. Time plus consistency will equal success. I'll say it again, Time + Consistence = Success

Not giving up: You can give up when you die. If you are suffering from being overweight, hating yourself, or any other ailment that brought you to this book, the key ingredient to success in life and in business is not giving up. And of course this all relates back to time and consistency.

Being in Tune: Knowing how to be in tune with your body is going to get you to your vision of success much quicker. Being in tune with your body takes time and repetition. The fitness community should be a place where everyone is able to just be themselves and not have to worry about other people's judgments.

Taking Measurements

"Doing exercise without monitoring yourself will be rare in the future of wearable technology." Astro Teller

We can't achieve the physique and health of our dreams by saying to ourselves on New Year's Day, "I'm gonna lose weight this year." That's a recipe for disaster. We can't expect to go anywhere without knowing where we want to go. For this purpose, think of our journey as a road trip. There are a few things we have to do before we can hit the road - check the tires, get some gas, maybe a tune up. We have to get some metrics.

None of the numbers we are going to collect matter in the end. What matters is the mirror. I don't even really count calories at this point. However, collecting data is going to help us to determine where we are during the progress of our recomposition. In the beginning everything must be written down. After a few months what you eat, how you train, whatever else you do will become second nature. Writing things down will force us to be accountable. After a while you will be able to eat and work out on feel. Your body will tell you what it needs once it starts becoming healthy.

Fitness Trackers

This is not a plug or a commercial to go and buy this product. In the world of health, exercise, spirituality, science, nutrition and anything to do with that lifestyle, it makes absolutely no sense to me why people who are active on a regular basis don't wear some piece of technology that monitors their vitals and their exercise statistics. Especially if you are trying to get in shape.

I have been wearing a Fitbit for three years. I have gone through five of them. I even keep all the dead ones stored in a Ziplock bag just because I am weird like that. There are Apple watches and a whole host of other companies that are in the game. I religiously monitor my calorie burn, my steps, knowing that if I hit 20k steps a day I have had enough exercise even if I didn't go to the gym, and I also record my sleep habits, checking every few weeks to see how often I am awake throughout the night and if I am getting enough deep sleep to repair my body and keep proper cognitive function.

I have had long discussions with people about wearables. One argument for not wearing them is that they are not often accurate. I have been wearing mine for more than three years and a wearable device gives me constant readings to use as a baseline. So even if it is not accurately telling me my calorie burn, it is giving me consistent numbers to work from. What I have found is that wearables are accurate and the statement above is just a myth. The early wearables were probably more inaccurate. If your smart watch is telling you that you have a daily average calorie burn of 3200 calories and you are eating let's say 3500 calories a day, that would be an example of one variable that would lead to your gaining weight. The same goes for if you are burning 3200 calories a day, eating 3200 calories a day, and gaining weight, then you know that your tracker might be off, and if you lower your daily caloric intake and start losing weight, then we know that how far off the tracker is. Wearables are also a good way to record specific workout types without actually having to write them down. The convenience of using an app to store your workouts is invaluable.

Calorie Counter App

There are a few good calorie counter apps available for your phone. I'm not going to plug a specific one as they pretty much all do the same thing, count your calories, but they are an invaluable tool when you are first starting out your journey to keep you accountable and to figure out what foods fit into your daily programing. I'm gonna be honest, if you are taking this diet thing seriously and eating five to seven meals a day, this form of accountability gets annoying. After six months to a year of steady adherence to it though, you will get a feel for what you can and can't eat throughout the day and that will make life a little easier. That is why I like fitness trackers. They are a tool that we don't really have to think about.

Three Key Physical Measurements

1. **Weight:** Although I hate using weight as a measurement tool this number plays a crucial role in giving us a starting point for reference. Even though it is not important in the end, I still have the bad habit of weighing myself multiple times a day. But the scale is nothing more than a tool in our bag. It provides no other benefits after we get in shape. You could be the same weight for an entire year, however your body composition may have been improving the entire time. The scale is a great tool for the initial phase of your body re-composition. If you don't have a scale please go out and purchase one. You can get one at Walmart for around 20 bucks.

2. **Body Fat:** Knowing our body fat is going to play a bigger role in our success. Body fat percentage is something I measured monthly until I had visible abs and only because I am crazy. I don't get my body fat tested anymore. As long as I have abs I am fine. When I started my weight loss journey, I was 36% body fat. Once I reached 10% I stopped overanalyzing this metric. And that's the point. We are just trying to get to normal. You can't maintain freak levels of low body fat and stay healthy for prolonged levels of time.

An example of why body fat is a greater measure of progress than weight is that the body can weigh the same amount, month after month, but have a totally different composition based off of what you are eating and how you are training. Food quality plays a bigger role than weight does in determining your look at the end of the day.

There are numerous ways to measure body fat. A very basic method would be to use skin calipers which pinch the skin or to use a DEXA scan (Dual-Energy X-Ray Absorptiometry) which exposes patients to x-ray beams of differing intensities. There are also scales which you can purchase or hand held devices which use a small electrical current to get their reading. All of these devices should be used as a tool to measure where you are at, not a sword to live by.

3. **Body Measurements:** In the beginning of your weight loss the biggest changes you are going to see are in your body's dimensions. When we first start exercising, our body is going to be constantly changing if we do everything right. We might even gain a little weight in the beginning as the body is freaking out a little. For our purpose, we will be measuring our waist, our thighs, chest, and arms monthly. We will be recording these numbers in our journal until we feel that it is not useful anymore. (I used to record my measurements monthly. I am less obsessive with this after years of progress. You will get like that too.)

Very Important Metrics To Keep In Mind

Basal Metabolic Rate (BMR)

Basal Metabolic Rate is super easy and important to understand. In short, our BMR is the amount of energy expended while we are at rest, the amount of energy we would use if we just sat on the couch and did nothing all day. Think of the calories that are used just to keep our brain on, make our heart beat, eyes blink, etc. Those calories. This is an important number through our entire physical transformation.

What is our BMR? Well, coincidentally there are many, ways to calculate it. When it comes to transforming our body there are a few accepted equations to calculate this number. These include: the revised Harris-Benedict equation; Mifflin-St Jeor Equation; Katch-McArdle equation; and the Cunningham equation. (Remember, at the end of the day, science is just an educated guess based off of using all the information at hand.)

Here is an easy **BMR** calculation if you are just getting started. For our purposes we are going to use a conservative estimate that it is going to take ten calories to maintain a pound of body weight.

So… Using me as an example 175 x 10 = 1750

That's about right. Prior to writing this, I had myself professionally tested for this book. The device we used stated that my BMR was roughly 1797 calories a day. Once again there is no exact number. We will only find the true number out through trial and error. However the 10 calorie rule is a great place to start for beginners. We are not here to make things complicated.

Lean Body Mass : LBM

Lean body mass is a very simple concept to grasp and is important for the next equation. LBM predicts energy expenditure. Think of all of your muscles, organs, and bones combined without the fat. Think of what that weighs. The idea behind our transformation is we are feeding ourselves according to our LBM which does not take into account fat. Hence the word LEAN. Through understanding how many calories we expend on a daily basis to support that specific mass, we cannot only control the rate of fat we burn, we can also put our bodies in a positive state to add muscle without spilling over too much and gaining an absurd amount of weight. This is equivalent to knowing how much gas you would need to get to a given destination. By understanding how much lean body mass we have, we can calculate appropriate calorie intake to achieve positive muscle gains. Cool, right?

To calculate your LBM, take your weight and multiply it by your body fat:
ME: 175 x 12% body fat = 21 pounds of fat, leaving me with a **LBM** of (175-21) = **154 pounds**

MY LEAN BODY MASS IN THIS EQUATION IS 154 POUNDS.

Please take a moment and calculate your LBM.

(LBS on scale # x body fat %) = Pounds of fat, leaving you with a **LBM** of (scale weight - calculation of fat) = **LBM pounds**.

Our goal is to feed the LBM based on our goals. And although it is not an exact science all of these numbers will put us in the right range for success. No one body is identical and what we are achieving is a guideline with these numbers.

So Joe, what do all these numbers have to do with our goals?

80

Good question. We are now at a point where we have some data to start designing our path to success. In the next section I am going to show you the Sterling-Pasmore Equation, the equation I use to achieve my goals and the goals of my clients. I have also modified it slightly so that it is a little easier to use.

Sterling-Pasmore (*SLIGHTLY MODIFIED*)

For all stages of your physical transformation I will advise that you learn the Sterling Pasmore Equation. Whether you want to get leaner or more muscular this equation will map out your caloric intake and give you an idea of your upper caloric intake for your goals. I like this particular equation because in order to be successful with it we need to be able to make an honest assessment of our activity level and where we are now.

This equation, which we will abbreviate to SPE, is the equation I have found to work best for me and my clients.

I'm gonna break down the equation and make it simple so that you can immediately implement it into your life (HENCE MODIFIED). In fact, I'm probably going to over simplify the equation. My goal is to convert all the scientific who ha into English for you.

Alright, this equation is based on our LBM. The goal of using this equation is to find out our **BESAL METABOLIC RATE** (BMR) including exercise expenditure. This number is the amount of calories we need in order to keep our LBM consistent based on energy expenditure.

In this equation the magic number is 13.8. **OUR THEORY IS THAT IT TAKES 13.8 CALORIES TO SUPPORT 1 POUND OF LEAN BODY MASS.** (Remember previously we used 10 calories per pound of weight. We are now using 13.8 calories per pound of **LEAN BODY MASS per Sterling-Pasmore.**)

So, if we use **154** as our example (from the previous LBM section):

154 pounds of LBM x 13.8 calories to maintain that mass = 2125.2 calorie **BMR.** Meaning the actual number to maintain bodyweight based on our level of body fat and leanness is 2125.2 calories per day.

For this example it takes 2125.2 calories for me to be alive and just function everyday. We have just figured out our true BMR based on our lean body mass. This is the amount of calories my body needs to go through all its processes. (Please calculate yours.)

Sterling-Pasmore states that once you calculate your BMR (2125.2), you then factor in your activity level to account for calories burned during such exercise. (This was the part I told you I was going to over simplify.)
So:

- BMR x 1.2 for lazy people and
- BMR x 1.2 for people new to working out (leisurely walking for 20-30 minutes up to 3 times a week)
- BMR x 1.6 for moderate exercise 3-5 days per week. (Remember 1.6)
- BMR x 1.725 for active individuals (exercising 6-7 days/week at moderate to high intensity)
- Theoretically these numbers can go higher based on your activity level, but I will assume you are not running triathlons yet or trying to become a 300 pound bodybuilder.

Remember 1.6? Well 1.6 is the number I use for my daily caloric intake. I workout 6 days a week, do 8 workouts, 4 of them being high intensity. In reality this number puts me at a slight deficit on a daily basis, but I am totally fine with that.

Ok. In our example my BMR was 2125.2 calories a day. With that said:

$$2125.2 \text{ x } 1.6 = \textbf{3400.32}$$

According to this equation and real life I need to eat around 3400 calories to maintain my 154 pounds of lean body mass at 175 pounds and 12% body fat based on the amount of exercise I do per day. If I want to gain weight I eat more than that. If I want to maintain my weight I eat right around that and if I want to lose weight I now have a starting point from which to cut calories. That is how we get to our starting point. That is how we map out our goals. I have found SPE to be a very accurate method of determining where we need to be caloric wise.

Please go ahead and calculate your daily caloric intake based on this equation.

Your BMR x (either 1.2, 1.6, 1.75) = Daily Caloric Intake

Now please remember that these numbers are not set in stone. For example, a number like 1.4 may work best for you. I choose to use 1.6 because I can slowly cut fat off of my body, while still being able to put small amounts of muscle on all while not being hungry and pretty much eating whatever I want. **3400** calories is a lot of calories to consume. I'm also able to go over or under a little and it is not the end of the world.

Food, Glorious Food, The Thermic Effect of Food

"First we eat, then we do everything else." M.F.K. Fisher

We all eat food. Most of us count calories. We all think about macro this and micro that and how many calories we are burning on a daily basis. But do we ever think about the calories that are being burnt for absolutely doing nothing? The Thermic Effect Of Food (TEF) or (Dietary Induced Thermogenesis) states that the act of eating will burn calories in itself. That is why the idea and concept of eating multiple times a day works so well for preventing hunger and creating a positive metabolic environment.

For every piece of food that we eat it takes calories to digest them. Energy is burned to extract energy from the foods we are consuming. Think of each meal as adding a log to a fire. With each log we add throughout the day, the flame gets a little hotter. It takes energy to digest food and after all, a calorie is just a measure of energy. The more often you eat, the more calories you burn.

The general idea is to eat as much as we can without putting fat on. We want to create an anabolic environment where we are just packing on muscle and burning fat as optimally as possible. Our goal is get our body to burn body fat as the primary source of energy as opposed to carbs. Or at least produce an environment where our metabolism has the opportunity to do that. With that said, we need to be aware of the type of macronutrients we are putting into our body and how many calories it takes to process them… roughly.

Fat, Protein, Carbs, these are staples of most people's diets, and, depending on our goals, we will be playing around with the ratio of each nutrient. In the end, regardless of what any doctor, coach, or expert tells you, it's going to take a little playing around and experimenting with your foods to see which ones work best for you and which ones don't. Very often foods affect people in different ways during the digestion process. For example, food X might cause discomfort and bloating for one individual and might not for the next. So where you get your macronutrients will take some playing around with, but the options are fairly simple and abundant. I'll also outline them below.

Fats and protein will always be a staple in our diet. In the 80's and 90's bodybuilders seemed to shy away from fat. They still had it in their diet, but the source was primarily from the large amounts of animal protein that they were eating. It's important to look at the nutritional programming used by bodybuilders and physique athletes. They are the ones pushing the envelope to the max. Over the last decade or so, athletes have realized that adding healthy fats to a program can provide dramatic benefits, especially when it comes to maintaining good hormone levels.

Carbs as we will learn are not the enemy. They are also not an essential nutrient and technically you could go your whole life without them. The ketogenic diet is an example of this and there are tens of thousands, if not more people, living a healthy life eating no carbohydrates at all for long periods of time. The keto diet has been proven to be very beneficial in treating patients with type 2 diabetes as well as various cancers. With ketogenic diets, lowering carbohydrates will reduce your levels of glucose, the fuel that feeds cancer cells. This will put your body into ketosis and will assist in depleting cancer cells of their energy supply. We, however, are not scared of carbs; we just understand their place in our nutrition program as a source of energy for rebuilding muscle and fueling workouts.

Fat is a vital nutrient for both men and women and is good as long as we eat the correct kinds. Monounsaturated fats play a vital role in hormone production, supporting healthy blood lipid and cholesterol levels and contributing to heart health.

Fish oil also lowers inflammation. And although our goal is to eat primarily healthy fats, specifically monounsaturated fats like avocados or macadamia nut oil, we are not going to shy away from saturated fats either, as they have been proven to support mood, well being, and overall hormone production as well. "Hey, who doesn't like a ribeye every now and again, right, big guy?"

Protein is the basis of all diets. If one thing can be agreed upon in the crazy world of diet fads it is that protein is essential. It can be considered our bricks on which we build the muscle, fat will be the mortar, and carbs will be the workers who build the wall (for lack of a better term, but to put it into modern context).

Of all the food categories, the digestion of proteins is the most time consuming. It takes between two and three hours to break down and digest proteins. The reason for this is fairly simple simple: proteins are chains of amino acids linked together. Some of these chains can contain thousands of amino acids and breaking them down requires the combination of good chewing, multiple bodily functions, and time.

Basic Macronutrient Breakdowns:

- **Fats:** Fats are an essential macronutrient. Our body will "use" 5% to 15% of the calories from the fat we consume to process that actual fat. Our main sources of fats will come from, preferably in this order, macadamia nut oil, organic avocado oil, and, even though it is low in monounsaturated fats, coconut oil because we want about 20 to 30% of our fats to come from saturated sources.

- **Protein:** Protein is another essential macronutrient that takes roughly 20% to 35% of the calories we

86

consume to process. Protein is essential in not only building muscle mass but also in maintaining it when we are trying to peel fat off our bodies. Our most preferred choices for protein would be red meat (grass fed), chicken or organic turkey, if possible, and white fish. Salmon, lamb, octopus, shrimp, anything that is ocean farmed sustainably is acceptable. Your staples are going to be beef, chicken, and fish. Mostly chicken.

- **Carbohydrates:** Carbs are super simple for our bodies to process and they can be stored in three places within the body. Carbs are stored in the muscle, as muscle glycogen. They are stored in the liver, as liver glycogen. And they are stored in the fat cells as body fat. They also work differently than fats. It takes about 5% to 15% of the energy consumed to process carbohydrates. It's undeniable that carbohydrates are an excellent source of energy, for fueling our workouts and in recovery. Acceptable carbohydrate sources are white rice, brown rice, quinoa, Ezekiel bread, sour dough (sparingly), an occasional bagel, all things in moderation.

Below are references to how many calories are burned approximately per nutrient consumed. (*And for this example we will use the maximum percentages that I referenced for you above*): Let's say:

FAT = 15%
1000 calories of **FAT** is consumed: **1000 x .15 = 150 calories burned to process.**
It will take 150 calories to burn the 1000 calories of fat we ate.

PROTEIN = 35%
1000 calories of PROTEIN is consumed: **1000 x .35 = 350 calories burned to process.**

It will take 350 calories to burn the 1000 calories of protein that we ate.

CARBOHYDRATES = 15%
1000 calories of **carbohydrates** is consumed: **1000 x .15 = 150 calories burned to process.**
It will take 150 calories to burn the 1000 calories of carbohydrates that we ate.

It is important to at least calculate these numbers once or twice as you could be missing out on calories that can add to your gains by thinking you are eating enough, but actually under consuming because you'd not take into the effect TEF.

In theory, diets like Atkins, and high carb diets that focus on having the "dieter" focus on one specific food group, make sense. These can be referred to as restriction diets or exclusion diets, which could be considered the same thing. However, what all these fad diets have in common is they don't discuss what is going on in our body while we are eating. They don't address insulin sensitivity, manipulating blood sugar levels, food timing, and putting these programs in place with specific exercise routines. My goal is to give you enough information in this book so that you can go out and develop your own ideas and hypothesis about diet, nutrition, fitness, and spirituality. I want you to go out into the world and create your own version.

Water

When I was at RedCliff, the wildness program, they had a tradition. If you were seen spilling a drop of water you had to recite the words, "Water is the essence of life. Water is the essence of life," indefinitely, until the counselor deemed you understood how important it was not to spill water.

Water is the essence of life and if you go without it for a few days you are a goner. In a healthy adult, up to 70% of bodyweight is comprised of fluid. Water provides lubrication and protection to organs and tissues and it maintains blood volume. The real question is how much water should we drink? That is dependent on your activity level, the environment you train in, your age, and what type of shape you are currently in right now.

If you are not in the practice of drinking water and are a soda drinker or tea drinker, it's crucial to get into the practice of having over 50% of your liquids, preferably 80%, to be pure water. That is my opinion. I drink about two gallons of water, a 32oz. coffee, and a can of diet root beer per day. That example is well over 80% water for all liquids consumed.

Most non athletes will be fine with just drinking glasses of water throughout the day when they are thirsty. In fact, this is my recommendation for everyone. Drink water when you are thirsty. Don't worry about having to drink a certain number of ounces or gallons. Just make sure as soon as you finish one bottle of water that you are refilling it. Letting the cycle continue each and everyday until the majority of what you drink is water.

I don't believe there is a such thing as "over hydration." I am constantly drinking water and peeing all day. The key to proper hydration is fully saturating all cells with good water each and every day.

It's important to understand that neglecting to adequately hydrate will lead you to dehydrate. Dehydration occurs when fluid exertion, including urinating, sweating, or exhaling, exceeds fluid intake. Fairly simple.

When there is a 1%-2% water loss in the body, strong thirst starts to arise. We start feeling uncomfortable, and we lose our appetite. From about 3%-5%, our mouth starts to become irritatingly dry, our skin becomes flushed, we have a decreased urine output and we start to become irritable. The next step after that is when we hit that 6%-8% range. Our body temperature rises and it refuses to decrease. Both our heart rate and our breathing rate cause us to become dizzy, leading to muscle weakness and slurred speak. (I like to call this Yoga Brain.) After that, it is basically bad news. We begin to have repeated muscle spasms, maybe some kidney failure, and decreased blood volume and pressure. I saw a guy in the locker room waiting for the shower pass out from being dehydrated. He hit his head on the floor and had to be wheeled out of the joint. Being dehydrated is bad news and we may not recognize it until it's too late.

Salt / Sodium

Salt and sodium are not the same thing. When people refer to salt they are usually referring to table salt, (NaCl), which is actually 40% sodium and 60% chloride. Most all salt that we are purchasing and consuming is sodium and chloride. Anyway if you read the word salt just know it is interchangeable to us as it will be referring to the salt that we eat.

Sodium or salt gets a pretty bad wrap. There is a lot of controversy on whether this mineral causes high blood pressure. Both camps make a valid argument, but I tend to lean towards salt being beneficial and not creating a high blood pressure epidemic. I myself am proof because I consume more salt than I ever did before.

If you avoid salt in your diet, I understand. I used to be one of those people, never adding salt to a meal, never really cooking with it except in limited amounts. But salt plays a crucial role in many of the body's functions.

If you are an athlete or just a normal person who lives an active lifestyle you can can benefit from an increase in sodium intake. Sodium plays a critical and active role in fluid balance, overall blood pressure maintenance, nervous system function, and muscle contractions.

Sodium is a positively charged electrolyte and, without getting too boring, it works directly with another important electrolyte, potassium. Together they play a vital role in fluid balance, regulating blood pressure, and the transmission of nerve signals.

The Food and Drug Administration recommends that the general population consume no more than 2,300 milligrams of sodium a day (about a teaspoon of table salt). I am going to recommend double that and if you are on the more active or bigger side, triple it. When I push my salt consumption to 5-7 grams a day my strength increases. I am less thirsty and I have no ill effects. I first started to experimenting with the 5-7 gram range after reading about it on many powerlifting forums. For more information on this you can YouTube: Stan Effering Sodium.

Potassium

Potassium deficiency is not something you really ever hear about and we will not touch on the subject very much. We are however including it as it plays a synergic role with sodium in the homeostasis of the body. If you are generally eating a clean dict you will be fine when it comes to your daily potassium intake. Most people are.

According to the National Institutes of Health Office of Dietary Supplements, "potassium is present in all body tissues and is required for normal cell function because of its role in maintaining intracellular fluid volume… Having a strong relationship with sodium, the main regulator of extracellular fluid volume, including plasma volume." ODS recommends 4700mg per day, but I would recommend going higher if you are increasing your sodium intake.

Why Do We Care About Water, Sodium, and Potassium?

Fluid balance is the key to a healthy body and staying hydrated before, during, and after our workout will ensure us peak performance both for our body and brain. If we are dehydrated, our body will have lower blood volume, reduced muscle contractions and we risk getting injured due to cramping. By consuming as much water as humanly possible throughout the day we will ensure that our body is able to carry enough electrolytes to help regulate nerve impulses and complete muscle contractions. Higher blood volume equals a higher saturation capacity for nutrients in the blood stream.

CHAPTER TWELVE
The Importance of Maintaining A Healthy Bodyweight and BMI

Throughout history, outbreaks of deadly diseases have decimated populations. In the Sixth Century, Constantinople (today's Istanbul, Turkey), was the capital of the Eastern Roman Empire. In the spring of 542 AD, the Plague of Justinian struck the entire area around the Mediterranean. Over 200 years, between 25 and 50 million people died. During the late Middle Ages, between late 1340 and 1400, Europe experienced the most deadly disease outbreak in its history when the "Black Death," the Bubonic plague, wiped out an estimated 200 million people. The last major plague recorded by the World Health Organization broke out in China and spread to India and was first documented in 1855. An estimated 12 million people died. So we know that plagues killed roughly 262 million people in those three events over the course of roughly 355 years. Pretty devastating.

In modern times, we may have avoided major epidemics, but obesity, very prevalent in today's society, is a plague and results in diseases that cost millions of lives.

It's very hard for people to look in the mirror and ask themselves if they are a good weight. If you are more muscular you are going to have a high BMI just like that of a fat person and the body does not really know the difference between a pound of fat and a pound of muscle when it comes to daily payload. For our purposes, we will look at BMI as a guide for being overweight or obese and we will use that word to define a sedentary lifestyle that promotes body fat distribution.

Heart disease, cancer, and stroke are all leading causes for death in the United States. All of these mortality statistics are directly affected by people being either overweight or obese.

A healthy body will fight cancer. A healthy body will fight fat. And a healthy body will create positive thoughts.

Obesity is a leading cause of preventable death across the globe. It is also a growing epidemic, and a major contributor to cardiovascular disease and mortality in the U.S. "It is frequently stated in scientific and lay literature that obesity causes about 300,000 deaths per year in the United States," according to the NIH's U.S. National Library of Medicine, "The increasing prevalence of obesity over the last two decades has generated considerable concerns about its health burdens."[1] 300,000 deaths are a lot of preventable deaths.

About 610,000 people die of heart disease in the United States every year. One in every four deaths is attributed to heart disease. Heart disease is caused by many factors, the obvious biggest one being genetics, being born with a good ticker or not, but high blood pressure, high cholesterol, and smoking are the three major key risk factors here when it comes to dying from this disease.

If we disregard smoking, as no one should be smoking cigarettes in 2019, and focus on high blood pressure and high cholesterol as major factors, we already know a few things. Having a poor diet is going to cause us to feel lethargic. If we are not eating the correct foods and too much of them, we are inevitably going to have high cholesterol and a myriad of problems created by the lack of clean eating.

This lack of proper nutrition in turn is going to enable us to make excuses as to why we are lacking physical activity. Once we get lazy we become overweight, leading us to become

---

[1] Flegal, Katherine M., PhD, Williamson, David F., PhD, Pamuk, Elsie R., PhD, Rosenberg, Harry M., PhD. "Estimating Deaths Attributable to Obesity in the United States." U.S. National Library of Medicine, National Institutes of Health. https://www.ncbi.nlm.nih.gov/pmc/articles/PMC1448478/ (11/2/2018)

obese and maybe even putting some gravy on top with Type 2 diabetes.

So, for conversation purposes, if we figure (loosely) that two-thirds of all heart disease is created from those factors mentioned above, leading to the high blood pressure and the high cholesterol, we can then claim another 400,000 deaths a year for being in poor shape. Do you see where I am going with this?

Next on our list are strokes. In the U.S., more than 140,000 people die each year from strokes. What causes strokes, you might ask? Well, you guessed it. The leading cause of strokes is hypertension or, as we were just talking about, high blood pressure. How does high blood pressure happen? Besides genetics, once again being overweight almost guarantees that you will have high blood pressure. Hypertension is another one that we won't talk about but it claims 410,000 American deaths annually.

High cholesterol is the next monster on our list. Having high cholesterol is going to promote the build up of plaque within your arteries, causing arteries to clog causing that fatal stroke. High cholesterol, aside from being predisposed because of genetics, is a direct result of poor nutrition education and making poor choices over a long period of time. Something that with practice can be corrected.

Diabetes is third on our list, but it's also important to understand its role in overall death throughout the U.S when related to a strokes. Diabetes damages nerve and blood vessels, weakening them or, in some cases, causing them to rupture. There are two types of diabetes type 1 and type 2. Type 2 can be considered a trophy for not taking care of yourself as it is totally preventable. A Harvard paper suggests that, "About 9 cases in 10 could be avoided by taking several simple steps: keeping weight under control, exercising more, eating a healthy diet, and not smoking." However, let us not downplay how many deaths this disease actually claims per year. Diabetes plays a direct and an indirect role for causing a staggering number of deaths in the United States each year.

Diabetes remains the seventh leading cause of death in the United States, with a total of 252,806 death certificates listing diabetes as an underlying or contributing cause of death in 2015.

According to Diabetes.org, "In 1980, the Centers for Disease Control and Prevention reported 5.53 million people in the United States with diabetes; in 2014, the most recent year for which statistics exist, that number jumped to 21.95 million people, a nearly 300 percent increase." Also stating that, "American life expectancy has been growing at a very slow rate for the past decade or so, even decreasing slightly in 2015. It hasn't yet been established statistically, but it's fairly likely that obesity and diabetes together are an important factor in this slowdown." It's pretty clear that it has been established statistically, I just don't think anyone wants to publish the findings.[2]

The last and craziest number I think out of all of them is that 38.4% of men and women will be diagnosed with cancer at some point during their lifetimes. Not half, but almost. Excess body weight leading to cancer causes about seven percent of cancer-related deaths, or 40,000 deaths each year out of all cancer deaths. Keeping the BMI out of the overweight to obese range is going to give you a massively lower chance of getting cancer.[3]

---

[2] diabetes.org. http://diabetes.org. (2/1/2019).

[3] "Does body weight affect cancer risk?" American Cancer Society. https://www.cancer.org/cancer/cancer-causes/diet-physical-activity/body-weight-and-cancer-risk/effects.html. (Accessed March 2, 2019.)

So what was the point of that Bubonic plague rant and you telling us about the leading causes of death in the United States? Well, if we add the numbers up starting with the biggest:

We have the 400,000 deaths that we estimated from heart disease. We then have another 300,000 directly preventable deaths from obesity alone We add 140,000 strokes deaths and then to that about 40,000 diabetes deaths a year.

If we add those numbers up without hypertension, which we already established is most definitely caused by being overweight, we get 880,000 deaths a year.
If we add in hypertension for shits and giggles we get 1,290,000 deaths a year. So to make things easy lets round the overall deaths based off our research to right around one million deaths a year from being out of shape, fat, and in poor health due to the nutritional choices we are making and then we have something to work with.

The plague reigned for a total of 355 years totaling 262 million deaths on the high side of history's recordings. By our estimations, if obesity was an epidemic for 355 years it would claim 355 million people in the same time with modest calculations. So my question to you, "Is obesity, the lack of caring for oneself spiritually, mentally, and maintaining a healthy bodyweight / BMI not an epidemic or plague of vast proportion? Is it not important to be mindful of everything we put into our body?

CHAPTER THIRTEEN
Fasting

No conversation about spirituality, enlightenment, and hacking the body would be complete without talking about fasting. In today's "order your dinner to your couch from the convenience of your thumb" society we are plagued by the overabundant accessibility of food paired with enough gadgets and doodads to take our attention away from ever hitting a gym or taking a walk around the block.

This has led the United States and, by way of export, the world to a development of unprecedented proportion. Every modern country now suffers from a plague of laziness and obesity brought on by the modern marvels of technology.

Today we can order food from a phone. We can order groceries from the internet and, if you are really adventurous, you can have them delivered to your car for pickup. Never really having to get out of your car, walk, even hunt or talk to someone for your food ever again. This amazing convenience has led to an unprecedented rate of disorders. In fact 75% of the country is overweight or obese. To be more specific, according to data from the National Health and Nutrition Examination Survey, "More than one in three adults are considered to be overweight. More than one in three adults are considered to be obese. Meaning more than two in three adults are considered to be overweight or obese.

Fasting is popular in today's diet market with many popular experts promoting "fasted cardio," "intermittent fasting," and various other fasts where you spend a large portion of the day without food. I'm going to explain fasting, but I am going to say over and over again... For our purposes athletically fasting is not necessarily beneficial to us as we will be doing daily physical exercise and will need food to recuperate. If we are trying to achieve spiritual benefits from fasting, that is a different subject which I will cover later in the chapter.

If we remember from the TEF section, the thermic effect of food, we want to be eating multiple small to medium sized meals a day in order to maintain a steady balance of nutrients in the body and to keep the metabolism firing all day. Our goal is to maintain peak performance for both mind and body and if we are not eating we just can't do that. Also as it has been stated it takes energy to extract energy out of the food we are eating so eating multiple meals a day is going to be beneficial for an optimal running metabolism. I will say it later in the chapter, but the only time I fast is from the time I go to bed to the time I wake up for breakfast.

Fasting is defined as a partial or total abstention from all foods, or a select abstention from prohibited foods. Fasting when used for non religious purposes in many cases is used as a potential non pharmacological intervention for improving health and increasing longevity. There also are numerous studies showing that living a calorie restricted lifestyle will extend your lifespan.

In recent studies conducted with overweight humans, caloric restriction has been shown to improve a number of health outcomes including improving insulin-sensitivity, which for our purposes, means we will store more nutrients as fuel rather than as fat. Caloric restriction will enhance mitochondrial function. Mitochondria are the energy factories of the cells. They take in nutrients, process them, and create energy rich molecules for every cell in the body. As an athlete, as a body hacker, as a human, this is all very important. Mitochondria produce ATP which is a complex organic chemical that provides energy to drive, muscle contraction, nerve impulses, and chemical synthesis throughout the body.

Additionally, prolonged caloric restriction has also been found to reduce oxidative damage to both DNA and RNA, meaning you live longer. The breakdown and damage of DNA and RNA are directly related to aging and many other negative health factors. Their findings of initial human clinical trials appear to support the promise of calorie restricted diets in adults.[1]

Fasting is a very popular fitness term used these days and, from time to time, it has a place in our practice for both spiritual and medical purposes. If you are trying to build muscle the only time you should be fasting is from the time you go to bed to the time you wake up.

For religious and spiritual purposes, fasting has been used by the Christians, the Muslims, the Jews, Native American Cultures, in India and the list goes on. Many of those cultures have taken it a step further and removed certain foods. Lent, Yom Kippur, and Ramadan are just a few holy days, out of many examples, where fasting is incorporated into religion. Virtually all schools of thought, religion, medicine, and dieting have incorporated fasting into their practices in some form or another.

For spiritual and religious purposes, fasting is to be used before and during special sacred times. This could be drug induced or otherwise. In some Native American cultures, fasting is practiced before a vision quest and during as a way of purifying oneself. In ancient civilizations, priests and priestess would fast in order to prepare themselves before presenting their gifts to their gods.

Fasting is considered an ascetic practice. That being said, it is usually reserved for times of intensive meditation enabling individuals to dissociate from the world and reach a transcendent state. Mahatma Gandhi survived 21 days of complete starvation and that's about how far the body can push itself

---

[1] Anton, Stephen, Leeuwenburgh, Christiaan. "Fasting or caloric restriction for Healthy Aging." U.S. Library of Medicine, National Institutes of Health. https://www.ncbi.nlm.nih.gov/pmc/articles/PMC3919445/. (2/14/2019).

without causing serious longterm and irretrievable damage, three weeks. Severe symptoms of starvation begin around 35-40 days, death usually occurring around 45 to 60 days.

If you are going to incorporate fasting into your body hacking, start off slow. If you are interested in experimenting with fasting, trial and error may reveal if you like it or not and to see if it provides you with any benefits. And possibly to see what all the hype is about?

I'll personally do a fast every month or so. If I am cleaning up my eating after a holiday or just a couple days after eating like crap, I try to do a 20 to 24 hour fast with just water and coffee. When I do use fasting, I use it more for general overall well-being as opposed to finding any spiritual or religious context out of it. It is more of a reset than a journey. Many times I am just feeling bloated and the easiest way to fix that is to start fresh.

I get great benefits from not eating carbs in the morning. I have a few feelings on this, one being that I don't really need any carbs or I need minimal carbs after sleeping as that is not a very energy intensive activity. However, we do need some carbs in our breakfast. Just way less than most people think. You could also try fasting from certain macronutrients from meal to meal or day to day to see how that impacts your performance.

To begin, I would recommend starting your fast by going to sleep. Don't worry about what you ate the day before, just know that when you go to bed you are turning off the pie hole. You will then have roughly eight hours of nothing to eat and not worry about because you are sleeping. Once you wake up, my suggestion is to stick it out for another 12 to 14 hours. For a first fast of 20 to 24 hours, you would be asleep for one-third of it. Throughout the day I would recommend drinking unlimited water, coffee, and unsweetened tea.

CHAPTER FOURTEEN
Carbohydrate Supercompensation

Enhancing athletic performance all the time.

Most gym experts, or people like me, when they are cheating on their diet will call it "carbo loading." We are going to try and do this as much as possible, but in a structured manner. What most people fail to understand is "carbo loading" or Glycogen "supercompensation" occurs only in muscles that were trained and in a depleted state. Only then is maximal uptake of carbohydrates possible with a rate of approximately 25 grams per hour for average adults and possibly 40 grams or more per hour for bodybuilders, powerlifters, and any other type of large muscular human. Carbohydrates are an important source of fuel for the body during physical activity and at rest. More carbs, more energy, more burn.

The glycogen "supercompensation" theory (achieving supraphysiological glycogen levels due to carbohydrate depletion followed by loading) was first theorized in 1967 in a paper by Bergström J, Hultman titled, "A study of the glycogen metabolism during exercise in man."[2] It was proposed that since aerobic endurance is directly related to the body's carbohydrate supply and rate of burn, that carbohydrate "supercompensation" could possibly have a performance enhancing effect in athletes and then they went and proved it.

Typically when a carbohydrate supplement is provided immediately after exercise, for our purposes within the hour, the rate of glycogen storage has generally been reported to be between 5g and 8g per hour for the meal immediately preceding the workout. Bergström and Saltin's paper studied the ef-

---

[2] Bergström, J., Hultman, E. "A Study of the Glycogen Metabolism during Exercise in Man." Scandinavian Journal of Clinical and Laboratory Investigation. https://www.tandfonline.com/doi/abs/10.3109/00365516709090629. (Accessed March 2, 2019)

fects of altering carbohydrate consumption for three days at a time and the results were remarkable.

After a period of three days of low carbohydrate intake (you can go four to be safe), the body is able to "supercompensate" for the lack of carbohydrates by taking in way more muscle glycogen than normal in the muscles that were trained. This is where full body workouts come in handy. The body when in a fully depleted state is capable of storing 25g to 40g of glycogen per hour. This is five times the amount of partitioning if you just ate the same modest amount of carbs every day. Day in and day out. Furthermore, we know from our own research, that coffee plays a direct role in the uptake of carbohydrates to muscles, somewhere to the effect of a 66% increase.

So for us, since we are trying to achieve peak mental and physical states of unity, this benefits us in many ways. Every gram of carbohydrate that we eat has the ability to store three grams of water. Since every gram of carb is stored with three grams of water we can expect "supercompensation" to increase the look and size of our muscles. If we are an endurance athlete this will benefit us as there is more energy for our competitions. As exercise up regulates the body's ability to store muscle glycogen, we can also expect to store considerably more glycogen than the 500 grams of glycogen mentioned earlier for the average human. This in turn is going to help us push ourselves further both mentally and physically in our workouts and competition.

How do we get the body to do this? When we are trying to achieve a "supercompensation" of glycogen in the muscles, we are going to do a full body vigorous workout multiple days in a row. You can super compensate specific body parts, but what I can't stress enough is that full body workouts through hot yoga are the best thing you can do for yourself.

In the studies, Bergström also had the athletes performing rowing and cycling, but we are taking it a step further and doing full body workouts exclusively. I recommend a full body workout because the "supercompensation" of glycogen is selective to only the muscles we depleted. By doing full body workouts like yoga we are ensuring that all of the muscles are being filled somewhat democratically. On top of physical exercise we will be manipulating the meals that we eat to better achieve this goal.

For most athletes a basic and simple way to achieve "supercompensation" is by doing three days of high protein extremely low carbohydrate meals. That would then be followed up with almost the same macro nutrient profile for protein and fats except this time it would be high protein and high carbs. On normal training days in an article in the International Journal of Sports Medicine, they recommend consuming a 1g/kg single feeding of carbs immediately after exercise and adding protein to enhance the insulin response. Glycogen replenishment is extremely rapid for six hours after high intensity exercise. So when depleted correctly "supercompensation" can occur in those days that follow our massive single feedings.

We can measure the degree of glycogen "supercompensation" by estimating the amount of weight we gained. Since each gram of glycogen is stored with three grams of water. If an athlete gained 2300 grams or roughly five pounds after a feeding, we know that an extra 575 grams of glycogen was stored. How? Well, simply put, 1 carb can hold 3 grams of water. So in an equation it would look like this.

$575 \times 4 = 2300$
or
575g carbs - 2300g of weight gained = 1725g of water

Since we know every gram of carbohydrate can carry roughy 3 grams of water:

1725g / 3 grams water = 575g
or
2300 / 4 = 575

If the body is holding five extra pounds after a successful "supercompensation," we can reverse engineer the math to show us that we were able to eat an extra 575g of carbs which led to another 1725g of water weight, which led to a miraculous weight gain of roughly five pounds. This is something that would greatly benefit any athlete that has to make weight then bulk up again or any athlete that is trying to manipulate how much energy their body can store say, for example, before a marathon.

To better achieve our goal, most of the carbohydrate consumption on day one of the high carbohydrate phase should be simple sugars and intake should not exceed 25 grams per hour or 75 grams every three hours. Carbohydrates should be consumed at least every three hours so that continual glycogen synthesis is occurring.[3]

In a study in the U.S. National Library of Medicine, subjects used only 10–15% of their muscle glycogen during 20 min of daily cycle exercise at 65% VO2 peak.[4] This is important because that study suggests that we can deplete our glycogen

[3] Prevost, Michael C. "Glycogen Supersompensation Enhances Athletic Performance." http://members.tripod.com/jpe_sportscience/Supercompensation.htm. (3/2019).

[4] Goforth, Harold W. Jr., Laurent, Didier, Prusaczk, William K., Schneider, Kevin E., Petersen, Kitt Falk, Shulman, Gerald I. "Effects of depletion exercise and light training on muscle glycogen supercompensation in men." U.S. Library of Medicine, National Institutes of Health. https://www.ncbi.nlm.nih.gov/pmc/articles/PMC2995524/ (3/2019).

stores completely within about 3.5 hours of strenuous exercise at only 65% of our VO2 max. VO_2 max is the maximum rate of oxygen consumption measured during exercise. So at 65% of our max we are running on completely empty and taping other sources of fuel between two hours and 15 minutes and three hours and 15 minutes into an endurance event operating at 65%. That is why it is important to eat during endurance events and monitor your fluids.

The above studies have also shown that the rate of glycogen resynthesis is also most optimal during the first 6 hours post exercise, and maximum resynthesis occurs when 1.5 g glucose/kg body wt is consumed during this period. The simplest way to achieve experimenting with this style of eating is with a three day on three day off protocol.

Sugar

Sugar gets a bad rap. Well, not really, but hear me out. The goal of our nutrition program is to burn fat, primarily when we are at rest, as opposed to carbs. We do that by tricking the body to burn fat instead of relying on sugar or carbohydrates. Or confusing the body with the goal of partitioning nutrients as optimally as possible. When we exercise we induce a rapid increase in the rate of glucose uptake in the contracting skeletal muscles. The key to sugar is to use it in moderation and to use it only when it can be most beneficial to your progress. Sugar's main benefit is that it is a fast digesting carbohydrate. This means it digests quickly and causes a rapid rise in blood sugar levels. Let's see why that is a positive.

The only benefit that sugar has to us is that by raising the blood sugar levels our body compensates by producing excessive amount of insulin, which in turn is used as a shuttle to force more nutrients, mainly glycogen, into our muscles. Insulin regulates the body's blood sugar levels and whether or not the extra glucose from food gets stored as fat or as energy the body doesn't care. It's up to us to help direct that partitioning and if we have depleted our carbohydrate stores correctly, our sugar meal will spare us from any fat storage, ideally.

The average person can store about 400 grams of glycogen in their muscles and 100 grams in their liver, give or take, depending on your size. After that, it starts getting stored as body fat. Obviously if you are a bigger human, you could store more and vice versa. Since one gram of carbohydrate contains four calories, the body can store approximately 2000 calories in the form of muscle and liver glycogen. It is also possible to manipulate glycogen stores, something that is extremely beneficial for virtually all athletes.

As far as sugar being good for anything else, it's not. There is, however, a plethora of mixed information out there and that's because sugar is big business. I have read articles from organizations that I respect stating that there is no direct link to obesity with the addition of excess sugars. Or that sugar does not play a part in the diabetes epidemic, but we are not stupid. We make our own decisions here. If anything can be proven relatively consistently it's that animal studies have shown significant overlap between the consumption of added sugars and its drug-like effects. Sugar addiction seems to be dependent on natural endogenous opioids that get released upon their consumption resulting in a flood of dopamine to the brain, giving us that feeling of pleasure.

In both animals and humans, the evidence and the literature shows substantial parallels between drugs of abuse and sugar. From the standpoint of brain neurochemistry and behavior research, the data is suggesting that the reward effect on the brain is the same. Have you ever seen someone nearly on the brink of orgasm when the waiter brings out the desert? It's crazy. I personally can get super high off a pint of ice cream.

CHAPTER FIFTEEN
Meditation - **Bridging the Gap Between Mind and Body**

"Meditation brings wisdom; lack of meditation leaves ignorance. Know well what leads you forward and what holds you back, and choose the path that leads to wisdom." Buddha

Everyone has multiple conversations, personalities, and emotions duking it out inside their head for the top feeling of the moment. That might sound a little strange at first, but is it safe to say there is an angry version of you upstairs, somewhere? Have you ever had thoughts of low self esteem come out of nowhere, telling yourself what the hell am I thinking? Have you ever acted not like yourself? Anger, shyness, self hatred, these are your multiple personalities that you have to deal with and it's normal. The key to meditation is quieting all of them down at the same time, whether involuntary or self induced, and then you will actually be able to hear what is really going on.

Have you ever been in the zone? A place where time slows down, where you have your best thoughts, and the creativity is flowing? Well, that is basically what meditation is - "the zone." Have you ever noticed when you exercise or take a long, long walk that you get into a flow state? You start thinking your best thoughts. Meditation helps us to remove ourselves from the hustle and bustle of our day and to work on another muscle, our brain. Meditation is like working out; in order to be good at it you have to practice. What we are practicing is clearing our mind.

Fitness, nutrition, journaling, reading, creating your life's work, these are all forms of meditation and can provide opportunities to get in the zone, or for lack of a better term "zone out," from the mundane busyness of life.

For our purposes, we are going to focus on the traditional definition of meditation which, for most people, is the lying on the floor version and clearing your thoughts method. Some people will advocate for sitting, but sitting can get pretty uncomfortable if you are doing it for long periods of time. That is why I advocate lying down and have used this method in airports as well as on the beach. It works pretty well. (Just put a hat over your face.)

So here are a few steps to get you started into a basic mediation mindset.

Step 1: Designate a place that you can lie down comfortably on. Ideally a yoga mat, but a rug or a blanket works. I have used a towel at the beach.

Step 2: Make this practice apart of your morning ritual or however it will fit into your lifestyle. (I suggest the morning as that is when I meditate.) Make it a point to meditate at the same time everyday.

Start small with 10-15 minutes once a day and as you get comfortable, instead of adding more time, go and attack your day. Add a second session later in the day. Twenty-minutes a session is the most I personally recommend, as we have shit to do. It would be great to sit crosslegged or lying down all day, but that is not a luxury that we all have.

Step 3: Set a timer on your phone. Don't be obsessive about the time, but set a friendly reminder that SNAPS you out of your thoughts. I like to be snapped out of my thoughts. As I mentioned in Step 2, I have stuff to do.

Step 4: To get into the meditation headspace, I will often read a passage from a book, set my intention for the day, or create a mantra to repeat or a question to ask while in outer space. For our purposes a good mantra to start with would be, "I am the man /woman. Or, today is going to be a good day." Just repeat that forever until your brain turns off. I have heard of people paying thousands of dollars for their mantras and that is just fucking crazy. It's your practice, make it that way.

Another method which I truly prefer is just siting down and focusing on my breath, in and out. Clearing my brain of any thoughts whatsoever, not repeating any mantra. Once your mind is fully clear you will be able to feel what is going on inside of you.

To do either of the methods above, we will focus on breathing in and out through our nose with a tight constriction in the back of our throats, making the sound of the ocean. In yoga this is called the ujjayi breath. Most people will choose to breathe through their nose and exhale through their mouth. I recommend doing whatever gets you into that state of mind. Meditating allows us to pull thoughts from parts of our brain that we don't normally have access to. It essentially turns off the busy parts of the brain so the other parts can speak.

Step 5: When your timer goes off and you are done meditating take a few normal breaths, look in the mirror and go dominate the day.

Above is a simple way to get your thoughts together through a relatively traditional means of meditation. It's not rocket science, however it does take some practice to get into the right headspace. Other activities that bring me to a more extrospective headspace are yoga, heavy weight lifting, journaling, walking long distances, and reading. All these activities produce a somewhat similar pattern of thought or "in the zone" moments.

And as a friendly reminder when meditating… Try not to fall asleep.

CHAPTER SIXTEEN
Crafting Your Routine

"Physical fitness can neither be achieved by wishful thinking nor outright purchase." Joseph Pilates

A good rule of thumb when transforming your body is to start small. Start by trying to stick to your daily caloric goals and don't push yourself at the gym to the point where you don't want to go back the next day. Over time you will get stronger, be able to eat more, and this will lead you to set new, more challenging goals throughout your journey. By starting small and not jumping into, for example, marathon training, we will ensure that we are setting ourselves up for success and not failure.

Exercise

Each and every year millions of people sign up for a gym, a yoga studio, or some other type of assembly place for fitness and virtually all of the people that actually stick with working out look the same year after year. Why is that? It's because the average Joe Blow or even intermediate weight loss health nut or enthusiast has a lack of nutritional education. To really be successful in achieving a strong, healthy, powerful body you must combine both nutritional discipline and exercise together. If you're trying to get to the enlightened headspace the cleaner and stronger your body is, the further you will be able to push it in your practice. However you choose to design it.

Physical and strenuous activity gives us the shape, metabolism, and the definition that we want. Also intense and physical exercise has a deeply spiritual and meditative like trance effect on people. This is not to say that you can't get to a normal or a decent body fat level without exercise, but what we are trying to achieve and discussing is mind and body oneness, synergy. That can only be achieved if the body is in peak condition or at least moving towards peak condition. Combining exercise and the correct eating plan will lead to faster and more sustainable fat loss than one or the other alone. It will also lead to a clearer mind.

Types Of Exercise To Achieve Our Goals

Aerobic Exercise vs Anaerobic Exercise

There are two type of exercise, aerobic and anaerobic and they are both going to play an integral part in our exercise programing. In the end, what you prefer is up to you, but there is a common misconception that aerobic exercise exclusively burns fat.

When doing aerobic exercise we are burning oxygen to access stored glycogen. The primary negative for us is that with aerobic exercise over time the body adapts, our aerobic capacity increases, and our body uses less fuel to do the same workouts. This results in us stalling out and explains why running does not always result in us losing weight. (I'm sure you have heard of the preverbal "gym plateau".)

Anaerobic Exercise

Anaerobic exercise is any physical exercise intense enough to cause lactic acid to form.[1] Anaerobic exercises are used to promote strength, speed, and power. It is also used by bodybuilders to build muscle mass. Muscle energy systems trained using anaerobic exercise develop differently, compared with those developed during aerobic exercise, leading to greater performances in short durations. High intensity activities, which last from mere seconds to up to about two minutes, are considered anaerobic activities. Any activity lasting longer than about two minutes has a larger aerobic metabolic component.

---

[1] "Exercise." Wikipedia. https://en.wikipedia.org/wiki/Exercise. (1/2019).

Anaerobic exercise exclusively uses glycogen as a fuel source as opposed to oxygen. Heavy weight training, sprinting, and any exercise that consists of short powerful exertions with high-intensity movements is an anaerobic exercise. I'm going to go ahead and tell you right now that yoga is both anaerobic and aerobic depending on the style you choose. That is why I am such a huge proponent of hot power yoga as a discipline for both physical and mental transformations.

Aerobic Exercise

Aerobic exercise can be low to moderately high intensity, but the difference is fairly simple. Instead of the body relying purely on carbohydrates and the conversion of them into glucose for energy, the body is using oxygen as the primary source of energy for the metabolism to function.

If we think of anaerobic exercise as exercise that makes us run out of breath and that we cannot sustain for long bouts of time, conversely we can think of aerobic exercise as stimulating the heart and breathing rate enough to promote stress, but in a way that can be sustained for long bouts of time. Running, spinning, the elliptical are all examples of aerobic activities.

In almost all programing, anaerobic and aerobic exercise will be coupled together for maximum results (for example: in a bootcamp or pilates class, or weight training one day and running the next). Our goal is to focus on both forms of exercise with a primary focus on anaerobic activities since that will teach our body to be constantly burning glucose and building muscle.

There is nothing wrong with aerobic activities and before the summer you will see me walking on the treadmill for an hour a day for a couple weeks before vacation time, but for our purposes cardio is for the birds. Our goal is to be in good shape year round with a healthy mind and body.

With aerobic activities the body adapts and becomes a more efficient machine. (This is not necessarily a negative if your goal is purely to become more efficient, but we are trying to create the ultimate being.) We want to be efficient, but we also want to be optimal. In turn, aerobic exercise creates a state where we end up burning less calories because of the fact we are so efficient, resulting in stalled progress or what some would call a plateau. That is not what we want or expect when we are busting our ass to get in shape. With anaerobic activity, such as weight training and yoga, we are building muscle which directly increases our metabolism.

In the end either method of activity will produce results, but anaerobic exercise is far superior to aerobic exercise when it comes to fat loss and that is what is going to make your life-style sustainable. More muscle means more fat loss.

HIIT

High-intensity interval training (HIIT) involves repeating short bouts of exercise for 30 seconds to four minutes with workloads near or above peak aerobic capacity. Training programs that include HIIT can produce large improvements in cardiorespiratory fitness and skeletal muscle. These robust gains occur within relatively shorter periods of time compared with moderate intensity or steady state continuous exercise.

Greater exercise intensity helps promote cardiorespiratory fitness, which is an important consideration for brain health given that higher cardiorespiratory fitness is associated with greater brain function. [2]

HIIT workouts provide improved athletic capacity and condition as well as improved glucose metabolism. Research has also shown that HIIT regimens produced significant reductions in the fat mass of the whole body. [3]

Power Of The Heat : Training In The Heat

Going to a hot yoga studio has almost ruined the chance of me doing any type of exercise that is not in an extremely hot environment ever again. It's part of the reason I only stick to the basics, bench, squat, deadlift, dips, and pull-ups when I go to the gym. Even in the dead of summer, I have to have full sweats on at the traditional gym.

When the body exerts itself to maximum effort during extremely stressful situations such as life events or extreme exercise it produces a set of proteins called "heat shock" proteins. There are numerous different types of heat shock proteins. For our purposes we will just be referring to HSP as a whole when we are discussing them, but there are two specific HSPs that I will discuss a little more in depth. Recent studies have also shown that heat shock proteins can be produced during other stresses including exposure to cold, UV light, and also during wound healing.

---

[2] Robinson, Matthew M., Lowe, Val J., Nair, Sreekumaran K. "Increased Brain Glucose Uptake After 12 Weeks of Aerobic High-Intensity Interval Training in Young and Older Adults." The Journal of Clinical Endocrinology & Metabolism. https://academic.oup.com/jcem/article/103/1/221/4565492. (11/2018).

[3] "High-intensity interval training." Wikipedia. https://en.wikipedia.org/wiki/High-intensity_interval_training. (11/2018).

HSPs are important for our goals because we want to produce an environment that makes these proteins available to our body at all times. HSPs are proven to benefit us in numerous ways. They play a vital role in transporting nutrients as well as healing our body. There are also some studies on how HSPs can increase one's lifespan.

To better understand what is going on here, let's first understand that HSPs are transport proteins. A transport protein is a protein that serves the function of moving other materials within an organism. With regards to HSPs they play an integral role in upgrading mitochondrial biogenesis which is a major adaptation of skeletal muscle to exercise training. Mitochondrial biogenesis, the synthesis of new mitochondria, is involved in the control of cell metabolism and it is well established that physical activity increases mitochondrial content in muscle. Mitochondrial biogenesis is increased, among other factors, by endurance exercise and caloric restriction. This is important because if you remember earlier we talked about how mitochondria is essentially the power plant of the cell.

Mitochondria is an organelle, which is a specialized structure that looks like a pill or a bean. We can basically think of it as the energy factory or the power plant of our cell. By increasing the content of our heat shock proteins we are then, theoretically, by way of involuntary action, increasing cell life through the production of more mitochondria.

HSP72 is one specific protein we will be focusing on. Increased HSP72 is associated with improved cellular survivability and tolerance to stressors. Through the same research, HSP72 was also found to prevent high fat diet induced glucose intolerance and skeletal muscle insulin resistance. HSP72 expression is markedly decreased in skeletal muscle of insulin resistant and type 2 diabetic patients. In addition, decreased levels of HSP72 correlate with insulin resistance and non-alcoholic fatty liver disease in livers from obese patients. This suggests that a targeted approach to exercise could increase your HSP72, thus resulting in the prevention and possible treatment of many of today's metabolic diseases.

For overweight or diabetic patients, or for anyone who wants a better quality of life with improved metabolic function, exercise elicits a number of metabolic adaptations and is a powerful tool in the prevention and treatment of insulin resistance. Exercise induced HSP release may also contribute to metabolic homeostasis by actively restoring HSP72 content in insulin tissues containing low levels of heat shock proteins. Meaning exercising in the right conditions can make your body normal. [4] HSP70 is another protein that scientist have found to play a housekeeping role within the cell. Exercise has been found to increase levels of HSP70 as well.

HSPs also play a critical role in muscle building. HSPs help to promote lean muscle mass by a process of chaperoning nutrients in the repair of cellular damage. This is where HSP70 comes in. In our case, post exercise, but this can apply to everyday life as well. HSPs do this by attracting amino acids to damaged cells and encourage them to convert into new muscle. HSPs also ensure that the proteins we recruit within the cell for new muscle fit properly and that new proteins form in the correct shape. They play a critical role in the repair of muscle. [5] In a recent study the US National Library of Medicine stated that, "Serum GH and prolactin in males exhibited a 16 fold increase when males were exposed to extreme dry heat one hour, twice a day, for seven days straight."

---

[4] Archer, Ashley E., Von Schulze, Alex T., Geiger, Paige C. "Exercise, heat shock proteins and insulin resistance." The Royal Society Publishing, Philosophical Transactions of the Royal Society B, Biological Sciences. https://royalsocietypublishing.org/doi/full/10.1098/rstb.2016.0529. (11/2018).

[5] Bell, Lee. "Heat Shock Proteins; Science's Secret to Muscle Building." https://breakingmuscle.co.uk/uk/fitness/heat-shock-proteins-sciences-secret-to-muscle-building. (11/2018).

[6] People are paying good money for their growth hormone and we just figured out how to increase it 16 times by jumping in the sauna on a regular basis. Pretty cool.

So it goes without saying exercising in the heat can be extremely beneficial.

[6] Leppäluoto, J., Huttunen, P., Hirvonen, J., Väänänen, A., Tuominen, M., Vuori, J. "Endocrine effects of repeated sauna bathing." National Institutes of Health, U.S. National Library of Medicine. (11/2018).

CHAPTER SEVENTEEN
Hot Yoga

After all is said and done, we will have yoga at the core of our physical and spiritual transformation. Every day if possible. Specifically hot yoga. Hot yoga in rooms resembling the heat of a pizza oven or the sun. That's a joke, but a good hot room is usually around 103 degrees and around 40%-50% humidity, almost hard to breathe. Note that a good instructor will gauge the room and use the fans and doors and purge accordingly.

Hot yoga, but yoga in general, will attract some eccentrics and damaged people, me being one of them. But this speaks to the enormous benefits that this 3000 year old practice has on self esteem.

A good hot yoga class is like any good drug, or a bad night of drinking. It will make or break you. It will bring you right up close to ecstasy, but probably closer to death, just through the physical exertion it takes to move your body around for an hour to an hour and half in a room with triple digit heat. It will force you to focus on your breath and your mind in order to stay in balance.

If you practice enough, if you do enough hot yoga, you will be able to go a little further into that abyss each time, hopefully coming back and getting a little stronger each and every day. That is what yoga is all about. In the right setting, with the right mood, it will clear all thoughts leaving you with only the curiosity of how great you can be. I have never left a yoga class feeling bad about myself. I have also never gotten bored of yoga as well.

Hot yoga provides a meditative and, definitely, if you go hard enough, a physical feeling of dying mixed with ecstasy and euphoria. It allows you over time (your practice) to be able to better control your state of mind in any circumstance. Because no matter what is going on in your life, no matter what is going on in your "career" you almost died in that class this morning and it felt pretty good! After a while, it could be a year it could be a lifetime, your practice will become less physical as your body adapts and that is when you will really be able to dive into the mental and spiritual benefits that a hot yoga practice provides. Yoga then becomes a way of life.

In life you have to be mentally strong, unattached, and always looking to improve yourself and others around you. Yoga allows you to do all of that. Hot yoga allows you to bring yourself to the precipice of death. Hot rooms are only one door away to an air-conditioned hallway (to quitting), but the discipline to stay in a hot room and focus on your heartbeat, and, more so, on your breath, enables and empowers us in our daily lives. The opportunity to quit is always present in class and in life.

There are no "tricks" to yoga. There are no "get good quick" schemes. There are only selfish movements to ourselves. Over time to we learn to control our breath, with that, our heartbeat, and then, our thoughts. If we break it down in it's simplest form, the mind is like a supercomputer and with its semi conductors it figures out where and how to distribute the energy. Think of the thoughts as chemicals that cause re-actions which are energy. Through our practice we learn to control our chemical thoughts almost like the act of blinking, it becomes involuntary.

Yoga is effective in the prevention, as well as in the manage-ment of stress and stress induced disorders. There are en-couraging results and studies that show promise with obses-sive compulsive disorder, depression, anger, and anxiety. Studies support the potential of yoga as a complementary treatment for all those listed above. I personally think of it as a primary treatment and prevention method for any ailment. It has been proven that yoga decreases anxiety, stress, and levels of cortisol. It does this by turning off our fight or flight response.[1]

---

[1] Kumar, Taneja Davendra "Yoga and Health" National Institutes of Health, U.S. National Library of Medicine, Indian Journal of Community Medicine, 2014, https://www.ncbi.nlm.nih.gov/pmc/articles/PMC4067931/. (7/2018).

CHAPTER EIGHTEEN
Manifesting

Don't get set into one form, adapt it and build your own, and let it grow, be like water. Empty your mind, be formless, shapeless — like water. Now you put water in a cup, it becomes the cup; You put water into a bottle it becomes the bottle; You put it in a teapot it becomes the teapot. Now water can flow or it can crash. Be water, my friend." Bruce Lee

I talk about obsessing, but that is the first step towards manifesting. There is, however, a clear difference between obsessing and manifesting. Think of the act of obsessing as attaching your feelings or expectations to a potential event or outcome that we want in our life and giving it no action.

Manifesting is removing all attachments to the outcome of a particular goal or situation, knowing that life can zig and zag, but living pure of heart and giving 100 percent to every moment and enjoying wherever the road takes you. Usually we end up at our goal; we just don't get there the way we thought.

Not obsessing on going left or right in a particular situation, but just going and trusting your true self, or "gut instinct" that you are doing the right thing. That is what manifesting is about and that is what self enlightenment is about, living in the moment. Getting back to your animal instinct, something many of us have lost sight of.

Here is an exercise I do everyday upon waking and it is now a reflex, just like opening my eyes when I come back to consciousness every morning...

There is only one step. I open my eyes and I count backwards from 10. (SO 10,9,8,7, blah blah blah...) I then say the first thing that I am thankful for that pops in to my head, usually my family, or my dog, because she is right there and then I immediately say something powerful and positive to myself about my future. For example, "You are going to help one million people better their lives within ten years." Or, "You are going to be successful."

Some days I can clearly see that happening, some days I can't. However I know that vision has been there for quite some time and I keep saying it to myself. And though it doesn't matter if I help ten people or a million through what I am doing, I know my intentions are inline with who I want to be.

Breaking that down even further. The goal of this book is to build great men and women providing superior guidance through my own trials and tribulations. The goal is to empower you the reader to be your own thinker and to design your own program or vision of success, at the same time not being a dick or pretentious about it. There are a lot of yogis and fitness experts that have this air of, "I'm better than you," in their step. We are not trying to go there. There's a lack of renaissance men and women in the world. We are aiming to be that and more.

CHAPTER NINETEEN
Sleep and Sleep Hacking

"I never sleep, 'cause sleep is the cousin of death"
NAS

Importance of Sleep

We pass out at night after a long day, the TV is faint in the background, our cellphone although it might be on vibrate, keeps going off, the light never seeming to fade. Even though we have paid a lot of money for these blinds, the streetlights seem to keep sneaking in and we can hear our dog from time to time drinking water. Current evidence supports the general recommendation for obtaining seven or more hours of sleep per night on a regular basis to promote optimal health among adults aged 18 to 60 years. It is also important to take note that individual variability in sleep need is influenced by genetic, behavioral, medical, and environmental factors.

Some of us are always tired and some of us would kill to get a decent night of sleep. Our circadian rhythms are controlled by the hypothalamus, which is a region of our brain, and the whole shebang is based on reacting to light or the lack thereof. It doesn't matter if this light is artificial or from the sun or if the darkness is replicated artificially. Our body responds to that stimulus by producing melatonin and blah blah blah. I'm not a sleep expert.

I use metrics. My Fitbit would be the best record of my sleep patterns over the past three years and it has looked like this. From January 1st, 2016 to December 31st, 2016, I averaged seven hours of sleep a night. From January 1st 2017 to December 31st, 2017, I averaged six hours and 42 minutes a night. And last year 2018, it dropped down to six hours and 18 minutes per night. A wearable also tells me how many minutes I have even been awake, in REM, in light sleep, and in deep sleep per night. This is important because we can also track our sleep patterns against a health benchmark of other wearable users.

There are a couple of things I can infer from my statistics. First, let me tell you I basically had the same job until the end of 2018. So for those three years I was working in an office. However, I was consistent with my diet and my exercise regimen through the entire time. This small sample goes back to the power of tracking your data and statistics over time so you can actually see the progress you are making. One day after a few years or few months you can see how everything is adding up. After reading my sleep patterns over the past three years I can see that I have been sleeping less and less each year. This could be because I am getting older, this could be because I am eating better, there is a whole host of factors, but one thing I can also see with my tracker is that I am also awake longer and longer each night for the same sample period.

Sleep is an essential behavior that takes up around one third of our life. That's why I feel it is important to experiment and find the least amount of sleep you can actually operate on. The US Centers for Disease Control and Prevention reports that 30% of workers in the United States sleep less than six hours a day. Just like the amount of calories varies from person to person, so does the amount of sleep. Remember, this is all based on daily activity and basal BMR.

It is important to talk about sleep loss because it causes a decline in mental and physical performance. It slows down recovery from workouts. It impairs memory, learning, metabolism, and immunity. Longterm sleep deprivation is going to lead to our body failing us. With that said we wouldn't be taking a complete look at the picture if we didn't look at the opposite.

Sleep Hacking

I'm a huge fan of sleep, but I have experimented with no sleep on various occasions both chemically assisted and non assisted. The longest I have gone without sleep was 2.5 days. I crashed right around noon the second day. At first I wasn't really sure why I was doing it. I think somewhere in high school I had heard that in 72 hours you will start to trip. I have also had random acts of insomnia where there was just no way in hell I was going to sleep no matter what I did and after about two days, I eventually passed out, waking up and feeling like a million bucks.

Sleep Restriction Therapy or SRT is actually a real thing. It can benefit anyone when performed correctly. SRT is a self-help method to retrain one's internal clock in order to reduce insomnia and is also being used to treat depression. The theory is that by starving yourself of sleep, your body will be forced to essentially restart itself. The University of Pennsylvania School of Medicine did a study where 50% of the depression patients receiving treatment were able to use SRT as an antidepressant alternative. I try to reset the system once to every two months. Experiment within your practice.

How to initiate a sleep hack? Fairly simple. Let's say you work a regular nine to five. You come home on a Friday night or you do this on a Saturday, it's up to you, and you don't go to sleep that night. The next morning you take your shower, go about your day like it's a normal day. Let's now say you usually go to bed around midnight, one, or two on any given day. Because you did not sleep the night before, you will find yourself falling into a much deeper and restful sleep earlier and easier than normal. It's that simple. No electrodes need to be attached to your brain or anything.

During the day where you are completely awake, try and keep your diet clean. Avoid anything high in sugar, as we don't want to have opportunities to crash. Feel free to drink all the diet soda, coffee and tea that you want. Needless to say you should not be driving or operating heavy machinery until you know how lack of sleep effects you.

CHAPTER TWENTY
Detoxification Diet Program

Once a year, I do a detox. I actually do this exact detox which is a variation from a detox that a famous bodybuilding coach gave me. I have made a few adjustments for the vegan, vegetarian or yogi so that we can apply it to our lifestyle, but the shell of it is simple and pretty much remains unchanged.

This program should be followed for two, preferably three, weeks. You must fast and this includes not drinking or eating for 12 hours a day. All of your meals need to be compacted into a 12 hour period, but hopefully after reading the section above you will be asleep for roughy seven or eight hours of them. You may, however, drink water, and this is encouraged, as much water as you humanly can outside of that 12 hour period, but nothing else.

During these weeks your body will be releasing toxins from your butt to your feet. Make sure you drink a lot of water. Alkalinized water is the best, however I understand it is extremely expensive for most people compared to the benefit of what you are getting.

You may also feel kinda weird at times or feel like you have to shit yourself randomly, but that means your body is working. A little pant shitting can be good for the character. Here's what you can and can't eat listed below:

LIQUIDS:
Water
Green Tea

FOODS TO AVOID:
No Diet Sodas
No Coffee
No Dairy
No Red Meat

No Wheat
No Eggs
No Protein Shakes
No Fruits
No Alcohol
No Cannabis
No Drugs
No Fried Food
Try to avoid artificial sweeteners if you can, but I know that is asking a lot.

DIET is three to four meals per day: one PROTEIN and one CARBOHYDRATE item per meal and as many vegetables as you can fit on the plate:
5oz protein and 40g carbs per meal (MEN)
4oz protein and 30g carbs per meal (WOMEN)

PROTEIN FOOD CHOICES:
White Fish
Chicken White Meat
Turkey White Meat
Tofu (only if you are vegetarian)

CARBOHYDRATE FOOD CHOICES:
Quinoa
White rice
Brown rice
Steel cut or instant oatmeal
Sweet potatoes
All vegetables

FAT CHOICES:
Macadamia Nut Oil, Coconut oil, or Extra Virgin Olive Oil
(Be careful there are reports that nearly 75% of the olive oil in the U.S. is fake or fraudulent.)

Braggs Apple Cider Vinegar. Take one tablespoon three times a day with a glass of water. This is going to help flush you out. Apple cider has also been studied for directly bene-fiting nutrient absorption, balancing the bodies PH levels, and improving digestion.

Raw cacao is a well known for it's antioxidant properties. Raw cacao is known to have 40 times the amount of antioxidants that blueberries do, be the highest plant source of iron, has more calcium than cow's milk, and is a natural mood elevator and anti-depressant. You can get a bag for around five bucks at the grocery store and you can pop a few in your mouth through the day.

CHAPTER TWENTY ONE
Substances to Hack the Mind and Body

"I inhaled frequently... That was the point." Barack Obama

Caffeine

"Recipe to recover more quickly from exercise: Finish workout, eat pasta, and wash down with five or six cups of strong coffee."
The American Physiological Society Press Release (July 1, 2008)

Quite possibly the world's most popular drug, caffeine. Studies have shown that caffeine by itself has the ability to increase athletic endurance by increasing the rate at which fatty acids are broken down within the body. Perfect for anyone who is aerobic or anaerobic training and looking to increase their fat burning. By utilizing fat as fuel this allows the body to spare glycogen. By delaying muscle glycogen depletion, the depletion of stored energy, endurance is extended.

Furthermore in a study performed by the The American Physiological Society they found that, "athletes who ingested caffeine with carbohydrate had 66% more glycogen in their muscles four hours after finishing intense, glycogen-depleting exercise, compared to when they consumed carbohydrate alone." Also, seeing the same benefits pre workout as well.

So drinking your protein and oatmeal shake post workout with a ton of coffee is actually going to steer the carbs away from fat storage and 66% more towards muscle glycogen storage. I personally would always want to have 66% more energy for the next day's workout.

The Mayo Clinic recommends up to 400 milligrams of caffeine a day. That appears to be safe for most healthy adults. It's equivalent to roughly the amount of caffeine in four cups of brewed coffee or 10 cans of soda. At 400mg you are probably going to feel pretty jacked up.

Cannabis

I can talk about the recreational benefits of cannabis for stress and anxiety management for days until I am blue in the face. However, you can read a million other books and blogs for that info. You could even go and smoke a joint and figure it out for yourself.

For the purposes of this book, we are going to focus on the benefits of cannabis for its use as a performance enhancing drug for weight loss and spirituality purposes. Cannabis is a psychoactive plant that contains more than 500 components, of which 113 cannabinoids have presently been identified. [1] We are specifically going to focus for this text on the benefits of cannabis use and its cannabinoids on the endocannabinoid system. I believe the plant should be consumed as a whole, as a flower. CBD has been gaining popularity for its medical effects, but THC can be upwards of 30% in a plant. I truly believe deep down that consuming the plant in its entirety leads to a synergistic effect with all 500 known chemicals. There is also a flood of questionable CBD hitting the markets from China. It can be sourced off of websites like Alibaba where the potency and quality is questionable, at best.

I have been an avid proponent of this drug for many, many years. Specifically, for its recreational and entrepreneurial uses when I was younger, but when I started my fat loss journey, totaling roughly 110 pounds, I used the substance for its weight loss and health benefits. None of which I specifically knew at the time. I just had an idea that if I got hungry, I would smoke instead of eat. It wasn't until I dove into the

---

[1] Lafaye, Genevieve. "Cannabis, cannabinoids, and health." National Institutes of Health, U.S. Library of Medicine. https://www.ncbi.nlm.nih.gov/pmc/articles/PMC5741114/. (12/2018)

subject and industry head first that I started to understand better what was going on inside my body.

"Wait! I thought that weed gave you the munchies?" It does and that's the point for some, but my anecdotal evidence and research has proven that just like when someone who doesn't need Adderall or Ritalin takes the drug, the opposite effect manifests itself. In this case, weight loss. However, cannabis is a natural remedy and its effects can be positive for everyone as you will read below.

So why is cannabis beneficial to humans? Coincidentally our body is completely saturated with cannabinoid receptors. In fact, our body produces its own cannabinoids which we refer to as endocannaboinoids, meaning from within and, in this particular situation, within the body. Cannabinoids are a diverse class of chemical compounds that occur naturally in the human body and the endocannabinoid system that has recently been recognized as an important modulatory system in humans that regulates the functions of the brain, endocrine, and immune tissues. The endocannaboinoid system is a long word for cannabinoid receptors. (Think of lock and key.) Cannabis contains phytocannabinoids, meaning cannabinoids that are produced by a plant. And just like endocannaboinoids which are produced within the body, cannabanoids are nothing but chemicals that produce reactions when they attach to the receptors in our body, inside the endocannabinoid system.

The endocanebanoid system, first identified in the late 1980's, consists of two receptors, the CB1 receptors, which are primarily located in the nervous system and brain, and the CB2 receptors, which are primarily found in the immune system, blood, bones, endocrine glands and reproductive organs.[2] The endocanebanoid system runs throughout your body. Coincidentally, recent studies have shown that the body produces its own cannabanoids, similar to that in structure of the psychoactive ingredient in cannabis THC or delta 9-tetrahydrocannabinol, THC and CBD being the two most known compounds in popular drug culture today. If you read that correctly, our body already produces chemicals that are almost identical in structure to the ones listed above. There are many many other cannabinoids that we know about but those won't be discussed in this book.

To further understand why I am talking about cannabis, we need to understand how this is important to our evolution as a human, specifically relating to fat loss.

Our country is fat and as examples of obesity continue to increase, the development of effective therapies is a high priority. Why not smoke pot to lose weight? As I have mentioned above, scientific studies are showing that the endocannabinoid system plays a major influence on the regulation of energy homeostasis, specifically on the CB1 receptor where endocannabinoids were shown to increase food intake. If the receptor, CB1, is blocked, the overall effect will be to decrease appetite and lipogenesis in white fat (fat burning).[3]

If our endocannabinoid system is hyperactive, we have an increase in fat storage and food intake causing us to be obese. Here's an example to give us an idea of what I am talking

---

[2] Pertwee, RG. "Pharmacology of cannabinoid CB1 and CB2 receptors." National Institutes of Health, U.S. National Library of Medicine. https://www.ncbi.nlm.nih.gov/pubmed/9336020. (11/2018).

[3] Horvath, Tamas L. "Endocannabinoids and the regulation of body fat: the smoke is clearing." The Journal of Clinical Investigation. https://www.jci.org/articles/view/19376?emulatemode=2. (11/2018)

about. By "taking a dose of CBD oil or smoking a CBD rich strain (which will typically bind with the CB2 receptor) we can inhibit our appetites, whereas a THC-rich strain can increase appetite because it binds more readily with the CB1 receptor. Hence, why you get "munchies" from certain strains of cannabis, but not from others.[4] Theoretically treating ourselves with CB1 antagonists (a substance that interferes with or inhibits a physiological action in this case CBD oil or CBD high strains) we can stimulate weight loss and improve lipid and glucose profiles, meaning the burning of energy which translates into the burning of fat.

Above was a brief summary on the benefit of cannabis for weight loss and by no means was an in depth article into the total benefits of the plant, but the summary is pretty simple. If you are overweight like I was, chemicals in cannabis specifically CBD are known to block the endocannabinoids produced by the body that make us overeat and store fat. CBD blocks the CB1 receptor from attaching to these natural cannabinoids, thus negating many negative effects of an overactive endocannabinoid system.

In today's weed economy you are mostly going to find high THC strains since that is what gets you high and commands top dollar at dispensaries. In my two decades of smoking cannabis and primarily only having access to high THC strains until legalization made it more accessible, I have found that a high THC strain can provide the same therapeutic benefits when it comes to appetite restriction, primarily sativas, like a strong Sour Diesel from Oregon.

Science is also way behind the human guinea pigs. With the advent of state legalization, the retardation of draconian drug laws, more and more scientific research is being done on this subject. Unfortunately, cannabis is still federally controlled,

---

[4] https://www.greenrelief.ca/blog/cannabinoid-receptors/ (3/2019)

making research funding limited in the United States. It is up to us, the outside thinkers, and now the Canadians[5], to help our fellow humans understand the benefits of this plant.

How to use Cannabis - or Any Other Psychoactive Drug - Spiritually

I'm not gonna waste your time and talk to you about how to inhale a joint. I am going to give you some tips on how to get the most bang for your buck and how not to fall into a hole of uneducated use. Cannabis as a spiritual tool is subjective, but legalization allows cannabis to be discussed maturely to an extent. To some medieval humans the topic would get you excused from the dinner table, but not our table.

I have put together some recommendations for using the drug for spirituality purposes. I am not going to discus whether the drug is safe because we know it is. We are going to discuss how to get the best experience from using cannabis. Below are some cannabis spirituality guidelines for anyone who might be interested or has never smoked pot before.

1. ABSTAIN

If you have never smoked cannabis before you can totally disregard #1. Although I do think it is important to mention that many people report not getting high the first time they smoke. I got ripped my first time and I remember that day more than the first time I fell in love. Some reasons for not getting high the first time could be not inhaling correctly, maybe not knowing you are high, or your brain might just be fighting, subconsciously, knowing it is not a normal state of being for you. If you are a habitual cannabis smoker, chances are being high is your baseline and you have built up a toler-

---

[5] https://en.wikipedia.org/wiki/Cannabis_in_Canada#Final_legalization

ance. Meaning you wake up, take one or many massive bong hits and go about your day. I don't necessarily think this is bad due to the positive effects we have spoken about with cannabinoid receptor saturation, but to reach the level of consciousness that we are talking about, a heavy smoker is going to need to abstain for at least three to four weeks. If I go a month without smoking I can tell a massive difference in the experience when I give it a go again at day 30.

2. KNOW YOUR TOLERANCE LEVEL

Know your tolerance level and go way past it. Growing up, we had a word we created when someone got too high. We would look at the person and laugh saying they were having a, "BWE, " a "Bad Weed Experience." For some of us, we thought this was impossible, but the truth of the matter was these people who were having BWEs were just freaking out that they were not in control. Some people equate that to being paranoid. With any drug if you feel like that, the trick is to ride that wave for the moment. Paranoia can cause even the seasoned smoker to think they are going to jail for smoking some chronic and eating a few mushrooms. That's just crazy.

At low levels of ingestion of prolonged habitual use, the user is in control of their experience with cannabis. It's almost not fun anymore. When you are a noob or your system is relatively free from THC after not smoking, you are much more easily able to have those experiences where the cannabis is in control and you are just experiencing the moment in all its infinite possibilities.

In January, 2019, I was driving back to Las Vegas after a recent cross country trip to the east coast to visit my family for the holidays. After not smoking for roughly 3.5 weeks, I decided to hit up a dispensary on the way back to Las Vegas while I was staying in a tiny house at the base of Pike's Peak Mountain in Cascade Colorado. Usually when I am at home in my day to day life, I would take a bong hit, do errands, go to the gym, get some coffee, a usual day. The cannabis in that scenario is part of my daily experience.

In Colorado, I rolled up a blunt, a Vanilla Dutch, with a strain I had never heard of before called Blue God. I made sure to stuff it with more pot than needed for four people, what you would call a fat blunt. I also don't smoke cigarettes anymore so the nicotine within the tobacco leaf is another guilty pleasure. I had started the day in North Carolina and by the time I arrived in Colorado it was dark and it was cold as fuck. I unpacked my bags, turned the heat up for when I got back and went outside.

After a period of abstinence, it's pretty normal for me to feel some sort of remorse, or guilt for getting high. I acknowledge those chemicals going on in my brain and I know where they come from. After all I was arrested for for smoking a joint as a kid and the rest is kinda history, wilderness school, etc. So I don't let that give me the preverbal BWE anymore.

Anyway as I spark up that blunt and inhale I decide to walk behind the shed as it was an extremely windy and cold night in Colorado. I am told those are typical. As I get to the back of the tiny house, which is literally six feet to my left, I end up looking down Pike's Peak highway in the dead of night and as I look up to the sky I can see Orion's Belt on one of the clearest nights I had seen since wilderness. I literally just stood there for 20 to 25 minutes in the dead cold of night, smoking my blunt looking at the stars and just thinking, "Man, how small we really are. Does anyone ever stop and consider that we are just on a rock moving five million miles a day in outer space? Literally all the shit I get anxiety over is nothing, a speck of sand, almost meaningless." That's what I would describe as letting the cannabis control the experience and I was only able to do that after a long period of abstinence.

3. INVITE AN INTENTION

You don't need to set an intention every time you take a bong hit, however you should be aware of why you are doing something habitually, that's a given. A ritual, like smoking, or waking up and telling yourself you are amazing, should be set before embarking on any spiritual quest, but we are not going to be going off on a quest every time we get high.

Most people just take a bong rip and, "Yeah, party on." I encourage you and suggest you think about whether it's about finding inner peace, doing soul-searching, quieting the thoughts inside, or connecting with a higher entity when you are consuming for spiritual purposes

4. PRACTICE AWARENESS

Any mind altering substance can lead us to question your nature and thoughts within our minds. Negative and positive thoughts may flood the brain at this time; embrace them, remember that they are just chemicals getting swished around in your head and learn from them, use them as a tool to guide you on this path of life.

5. IT'S MEDICINE

Make yourself comfortable, don't overthink it. Allow the drug to teach you what you need to know and decide if it's something you need in your life. In most states cannabis is recreational so there should be no shame in going to the dispensary on a Friday night, getting a bag of weed, putting a movie on and seeing what happens.

When using any drug, be it psychoactive drugs or even antibiotics, always ask yourself if what you are doing is serving the purpose you need it to in the way you intended it for. If smoking pot or doing psychedelics from time to time is not for you, let it go. It's not part of your journey. If the effects of THC are too strong, remember there are weaker strains and there are also strains high in CBD with no THC that you can experiment with. Responsibility is the key.

Psilocybin and LSD for Depression

"Whether the mushroom came from outer space or not, the presence of psychedelic substances in the diet of early human beings created a number of changes in our evolutionary situation. When a person takes small amounts of psilocybin visual acuity improves. We can actually see better, and this means that the animals allowing psilocybin into their food chain would have increased hunting success, which means increased food supply, which means increased reproductive success, which is the name of the game in evolution." Terrence McKenna

In Paul Stamet's book, he writes, "Humanities use of mushrooms extends back to the Paleolithic times. Few people, even anthropologists, comprehend how influential mushrooms have been in affecting the course of human evolution. They have played pivotal roles in ancient Greece, India, and Mesoamerica. True to their beguiling nature, fungi have always elicited deep emotion responses: from adulation to those who understand them to outright fear by those who do not."

Besides obesity, depression is one of the fastest growing health problems we face today. And an even more controversial subject relating to health and fitness, is the use of psychedelics and their mind altering benefits to alleviate said depression.

I remember growing up and hearing the old wive's tale that if you have tripped more than 20 times you are legally insane. Or the man who walked out into the rain with a sheet of blotter paper and turned into a glass of orange juice. All stories, of course, being propaganda from the Reefer Madness age.

Psilocybin or magic mushrooms have been around since the advent of humanity. For thousands of years, native cultures throughout the world have experimented with small doses of this fungi for its healing and spiritual benefits. In fact, it is legal to posses the non dried mushroom in New Mexico and in recent times this food, the mushroom, has been gaining more popularity as an anti depressive alternative to prescription medication.

In 2018 the FDA gave psilocybin "breakthrough therapy" designation to a company called Compass Pathways for the potential therapy of treatment-resistant depression. Compass is now allowed to test magic mushrooms on people where all other forms of treatment have failed.

When a drug is given breakthrough therapy designation, this signifies that there is enough preliminary clinical evidence showing and demonstrating substantial improvement over available therapies and drugs. The breakthrough therapy designation is also designed to expedite the development and review of drugs that are intended to treat serious conditions.

This designation could be interpreted as a strong endorsement by the FDA for the potential of psilocybin therapy in the future. It also allows for many more clinical trials to be performed so that suffering caused by mental illness can be alleviated.

As we have already established, I'm a firm believer that physical exercise, the act of exerting yourself in a strenuous manner, will alleviate all of the body's ailments, but for those of us who do not choose physical exertion and seek western medicine's answers there are 100 million people around the world who do not respond to existing treatments.

Currently there are two states proposing recreational legalization of psilocybin mushrooms on their bill's for the year 2020, California and, most recently, Oregon. If that does happen, there will be more funding and more opportunities to study this natural herbal remedy without the stigma of being a hard drug user. Most recently Denver decriminalized the possession of magic mushrooms as well.

Here's some food for thought. Have you ever notices that all the fun drugs are schedule 1 with the exception of heroin and all the prescription and shitty drugs made it to schedule 2?

If you ever have a chance, Google the stoned ape theory of evolution. In short, Terence McKenna one of the fathers of modern human awareness, equated mushrooms to the "evolutionary catalyst" from which language, projective imagination, the arts, religion, philosophy, science, and all of human culture sprang. In short, monkeys ate magic mushrooms and started thinking outside the box. And while we will truly never know if this theory is correct, please email me after your first trip.

It's important to know again that at low doses mushrooms will improve visual acuity by increasing single edge detection. At slightly higher doses sexual arousal is present and everything that falls under arousal of the central nervous system, which is a factor that would produce reproductive success) and at extremely high doses both religious, spiritual, and mystical experiences have been reported.[6]

LSD or lysergic acid diethylamide is a synthetic psychoactive compound that was first created in 1938 by Albert Hofmann. In fact, its psychedelic properties were discovered by mistake when Hoffman took a dose of 250 micrograms, which coin-

---

[6] Mandrake, Dr. K., Haze, Virginia. "The Psilocybin Mushroon Bible: The Defibitive Guide to Growing and Using Magic Mushrooms." Green Candy Press.

cidentally he thought was the threshold dose. Turns out the actual threshold to feel LSD is 20 micrograms. Hoffman is known for his famous bicycle ride where he got home and thought he was going crazy, calling the doctor, not having any symptoms except dilated pupils. Later Hoffman journaled that after his terror subsided (his BWE) that, "I was able to enjoy the unprecedented colors and plays of shapes that persisted behind my closed eyes. Kaleidoscopic, fantastic images surged in on me, alternating, variegated, opening and then closing themselves in circles and spirals, exploding in colored fountains, rearranging and hybridizing themselves in constant flux ..."[7]

In the 1950's and 60's LSD was sold as a medication to treat depression, anxiety, and drug dependence. It was a widely used medicine with positive preliminary results. However, due to the counter culture revolution of the 60's, this drug was made illegal and is extremely hard to obtain.

Both LSD and psilocybin have extremely similar chemical structures with psilocybin lasting roughly four to six hours and LSD as long as 12-16. Each drug acting like the other and considered an entheogen, or a substance that can be the catalyst to spiritual out of body experiences when taken in large doses. When used in the proper setting these compounds are very safe. LSD is more of an energetic experience where as mushrooms provide a more relaxed trip.

For our needs we will be discussing micro dosing, which over the last decade, has become an popular method of ingesting these drugs. For those of you who don't know, micro dosing is the act of taking a substance in small quantities. Quantities which are low enough to not effect the whole body, but still

---

[7] https://en.wikipedia.org/wiki/History_of_lysergic_acid_diethylamide#"Bicycle_Day"(3/2019)

large enough to produce cellular effects.[8] The idea is we get the benefits of the substance without the recreational mind bending visuals.

What are the benefits of micro dosing magic mushrooms or LSD? Since both of these drugs are Schedule 1 drugs which the government annotates as items with high potential for abuse, we have to look once again to the human guinea pigs. In this case we will refer to the nerds in Silicon Valley who have been experimenting with this idea for quite some time now. Both mushrooms and LSD have been proven to treat depression, anxiety, helping with brain repair and cell growth, but more recently are being used for productivity. [9] With a micro dose you can still operate all of your basic functions of daily life. The effects can be so subtle that you may not even notice that it's there. This "sub-perceptual" dose is just enough to experience the myriad of benefits these drugs have to offer, but not enough to have a "psychedelic" experience.[10]

At any dose of these drugs, the body quickly gets to work at metabolizing each chemical. Once the LSD or psilocybin is metabolized, psilocybin is considered a pro drug which is inactive and needs to be converted into psilocin in order for us to get high, it can then bind to our serotonin receptors. Research is currently suggesting that we "trip" because the brain is becoming hyper connected and allowing greater communi-

---

[8] "Microdosing." Wikipedia. https://en.wikipedia.org/wiki/Microdosing. (12/2018).

[9] Kuchler, Hannah. "How Silicon Valley rediscovered LSD." Financial Times, August 10, 2017. https://app.ft.com/content/0a5a4404-7c8e-11e7-ab01-a13271d1ee9c. (12/2018.)

[10] Glatter, Robert, MD. "LSD Microdosing: The New Job Enhancer in Silicon Valley and Beyond?" Forbes, Nov. 27, 2015. https://www.forbes.com/sites/robertglatter/2015/11/27/lsd-microdosing-the-new-job-enhancer-in-silicon-valley-and-beyond/#497c51a3188a. (12/2018).

cation between parts of the brain that don't normally talk. Altered senses of sound, sense of self, space, time and colors are prevalent with both drugs since they are so similar in chemical structure. Both resemble the chemical serotonin and mimic its actions. [11]

What is a micro dose of each drug? Since tolerance to psychedelics build up rather quickly, it is recommended with mushrooms that you start with .25 of a gram or a smaller dose and move up from there. With LSD the general consensus is 10-15 micrograms.

Each human will vary in their dosages, but one thing is for certain... If you are going to experiment on yourself in this manner starting with less is more. From personal experience mushrooms are not very intimidating and easier to dose since you can use a scale. They can make you feel like a baby, helpless, introspective, and humble, with the effect wearing off in roughly six hours.

LSD usually comes on a piece of paper or in liquid form. With that said the dosing for a paper tab is a little harder to manipulate. Most users will take a 100 microgram tab (piece of paper) or one drop of LSD liquid and mix it into a one ml solution of bacteriostatic water, producing ten microgram dosages that would be divided out by a dropper.

Once again it has to be said, I do not condone the use of illegal narcotics, however I do believe that if you are going to experiment you should know what you are getting into and you should be extremely educated on what the potential dangers might be. I also recommend have a sitter, or someone with you for your first time in case you do have a negative reaction.

---

[11] Mandrake, Dr. K., Haze, Virginia. "The Psilocybin Mushroom Bible: The Definitive Guide to Growing and Using Magic Mushrooms." Green Candy Press.

DMT

N,N-Dimethyltryptamine or DMT is an extremely powerful psychedelic that gives you a short, but intense journey into a multidimensional, out-of-body, geometric, experience. It was synthesized in 1956 by Hungarian chemist, Stephen Szara, and is naturally produced in the body, but since then it has baffled both users and researchers alike.

Famously dubbed "the spirit molecule" by Dr. Rick Strassman, who, coincidentally tested this substance on people for long periods of time through IV, stated that this tryptamine alkaloid produces an intense psychedelic experience when ingested, and appears in trace amounts in human blood and urine, suggesting it must be produced within the body. The purpose it serves, however, remains a mystery. Users describe being transported to a distant realm where they meet seemingly autonomous entities. [12]

In his research Strassman theorized that we produce DMT for use when we sleep, explaining the imagery of our dreams and giving a potential explanation of the white light that is reported with near death experiences.

Low doses (0.05 to 0.1 mg/kg) of DMT primarily affect physical and emotional states with few to no perceptual hallucinations. However higher doses typically produce a rapidly moving kaleidoscopic display of intensely "techno-colored" imagery. Many people have reported ingesting DMT and meeting "other beings" in such realm. McKenna named this place the dome, the first archetypal location that he acknowledges. Many people find themselves in this domed, usually

---

[12] Taub, Benjamin. "Do Our Brains Produce DMT, And If So, Why?" Beckley Foundation. https://beckleyfoundation.org/2017/07/05/do-our-brains-produce-dmt-and-if-so-why/. (1/2019).

subterranean, place characterized by its jeweled, geodesic, and fractalized qualities. [13]

Ayahuasca

Ayahuasca is entheogenic brew used for centuries by indigenous tribes for spiritual and medical purposes and is now become a popular western remedy, for things like addiction, depression, and suicidal thoughts.

The ayahuasca tea contains two separate plants *B. capii* and *P. viridis*. The *B. capii* plant contains the MAOIs that allow DMT to have its psychoactive effects and these MAOIs include harmine, tetrahydroharmine (THH), and harmaline, although other alkaloids are also present. The *P. viridis* plant contains the single major hallucinogenic alkaloid, DMT. Together they create an experience which can last up to half a day with the entirety of the experience lasting your life. Ayahuasca experiences are said to be extremely profound and life changing. Many users report visual, auditory, and emotional changes through the experience that come in waves. This medicine is best administered by a shaman. If you are curious about a Ayahyasca experience there are places in the U.S. that will provide the service. However, if you are really interested in a traditional ceremony, you can google ayahuasca retreats and a multitude of sources will appear to you.

Anabolic and Androgenic Compounds

Performance enhancing drugs are a controversial subject, albeit a necessary one to discuss in a day and age where your favorite baseball player, cyclist, olympic athlete, and, most recently, an MMA fighter, are denying their drug use. A book about hacking the body wouldn't be complete without dis-

---

[13]Gaia Staff. "Scientists Want to Know More About DMT Entities People Encounter." Gaia. https://www.gaia.com/article/people-meet-dmt-entities-researchers-want-know-more. (1/2019).

cussing the controversial subject of PED's or performance enhancing drugs. (Needless to say, two of the items below, testosterone and deca durabolin, should NEVER be used by a female body hacker.)

I'll say it again. As a body hacker we are engaged in altering our system features to accomplish a goal that differs from the original purpose of the system. Hacking's definition refers to non-malicious activities involving unusual or improvised alterations to equipment, processes, and systems and that is what we are doing to achieve our goals. Our goal is to improve the system that we are living in. As the body gets older it deteriorates and with intelligent use of PED's we can slow down and sometimes even negate this from happening.

For our purposes the main benefit of these drugs is increased recovery time and increased nutrient absorption. That is all we want when building muscle. And as always if you are not putting in the hard work, you will not receive the maximum benefits from these substances.

I would truly be doing a disservice to you the reader if I didn't include this subject, but instead decided to lie to you and state that it is rare in today's society that anyone uses these compounds. In fact, once the eye is trained or once you have experience with these chemicals, it would be almost ignorant to not believe that even the average weekend warrior gym rat is not using such compounds, especially when they are cheaper than 90 percent of the products you purchase in the supplement store. It is inevitable in today's society that you will have access to these compounds at some point in your journey. That is why we must be educated in their use. Needless to say results come from nutrition, cardio, rest, then, if you choose, drugs. (Drugs are truly optional in your journey. I would never advocate someone breaking the law.)

It would be ignorant to acknowledge or deny that these substances don't work and work well when used in an educated manner. In fact, when used correctly, in moderation with an educated mind and under a doctor's supervision, the argument could be made that that these substances are safer than alcohol, cigarettes, and many of the recreational party drugs that society is using today. Below we are going to discuss a few chemicals substances. Once again I highly suggest not going down this route, but if you do please be as honest and forthright with your doctor as you have patient doctor confidentially.

There are three types of therapy that I want to talk about. TRT / HRT, Bodybuilding Dosages, and functional muscle / athletic performance dosages, but first we must understand what compounds we are talking about and how they work. All of the substances below can be obtained from a licensed physician. The only way that I would condone this use is when prescribed by a doctor. Obtaining these drugs is very easy when you have health insurance.

Testosterone

Testosterone is what makes men. It gives them their characteristic deep voices, large muscles, facial and body hair, distinguishing them from women. It stimulates the growth of the genitals at puberty, plays a role in sperm production, fuels libido, and contributes to normal erections. It also fosters the production of red blood cells, boosts mood, and aids cognition.[14]

For the purposes of this book we will focus on testosterone, deca-durobolin, and HGH since they are obtainable (if you have money) with a doctor's prescription, but I will also

---

[14] Ferrari, Nancy. "A Harvard experts shares his thoughts on testosterone-replacement therapy." Harvard Health Publishing, Harvard Medical School. https://www.health.harvard.edu/blog/a-harvard-expert-shares-his-thoughts-on-testosterone-replacement-therapy-2009031141. (11/2018).

briefly describe some other compounds and how they relate to body hacking.

Testosterone is produced naturally within all humans, most animal species, and it is even found in plants. The vast majority of prescription testosterone (cream, gel, injectable, patch, subcutaneous, etc.) are derived from plant sources such as soybeans and yams. It is considered the safest anabolic steroid one could use for this reason, due to the fact that it is the hormone that each individual's body already produces and already uses. Therefore, the use of Testosterone for the purpose of performance and physique enhancement is simply the equivalent of introducing more of a hormone into the human body that it already manufactures and uses.

When prescribed by a doctor for testosterone replacement therapy (TRT) or hormone replacement therapy (HRT) dosages will range from 100mg to 200mg of Testosterone Cypionate every two to four weeks. [15]

However, even as a non Harvard graduate with a little research, we can see that the half-life is roughly eight days which means that the peak concentration in your blood is halved at about day eight. So if you had a 100mg shot, by day 16 you would only be running on 50mg, by day 24 you would have 25mg in your system. This leads to very uneven blood levels. For the athlete, body hacker, and even to a degree a prescribed patient, these are very very low amounts of testosterone to have in the body after day eight and somewhat insufficient. By day 16, this amount of testosterone in your body would be insignificant and barely able to produce anything but a hard on and even that is debatable.

———————————————

[15] Ferrari, Nancy. "A Harvard experts shares his thoughts on testosterone-replacement therapy." Harvard Health Publishing, Harvard Medical School. (11/2018). https://www.health.harvard.edu/blog/a-harvard-expert-shares-his-thoughts-on-testosterone-replacement-therapy-2009031141

To give you an opposite view of the spectrum, bodybuilders will use anywhere from 1000mg to 3000mg a week, meaning 15 times the amount of testosterone prescribed by a doctor. And while these numbers are absolutely insane, these guys are the pioneers of physical body hacking and we can learn a lot from both their success and more so from their mistakes. With dosages like that injections would have to be done anywhere from three to four times a week. Now we are talking about health and fitness and without talking about the side effects of these dosages just yet, let's talk about the heart. Being 300 pounds whether you are a bodybuilder or a fat ass is not healthy. Your heart does not know if you are jacked. All that it is aware of is that it has to pump blood to 300 pounds of mass. Frequency of injection and dosage aside, this is not a healthy game plan for the body hacker.

And that leads us to the athletic dosage, the dosage that your favorite athlete, Instagram model, or fitness star is taking. If you do not think that most every fitness professional on the planet has taken some sort of PED in their career or is on some sort of PED at the moment you are being naive and not living in 2019. Our country prides itself on the superhero and action star look. Would you have watched the *Predator* or *Rocky* if the star looked like PeeWee Herman or Gumby? I think not.

Let's put aside the cheating aspect. This book is not centered or aimed at the professional athlete. It is designed to help the average human achieve peak levels of transformation and self enlightenment. With that said the average reader of this book will not be cheating at anything only enhancing their mind, body, and quality of life.

The issue here is not whether or not you think this is moral. Drugs work, that is why you go to the doctor for a prescription when you are sick. By doing your research, educating yourself and using substances in moderation we are able to achieve our goals faster, with less overall damage to our body. After all, the act of working out is to break down the muscles, producing damage. The rest periods are when the body grows. The use of PED's enables us to repair the body at a faster rate than we could naturally.

For athletes, we now understand that the prescribed dose by doctors is insufficient for performance enhancing because as we have learned this can lead to unstable blood plasma concentration levels of testosterone in our body. And we don't want to take these crazy physiological doses that bodybuilders take because we want to have functional muscle and still remain healthy, meaning we want muscle that will adapt and benefit us in the sport of our choosing and lifestyle that we are living. This brings us to the athletic dosage.

Athletic dosages will promote increased muscle building, increased recovery time and increased nutrient absorption. That is all we want out of our PEDs, the ability to hit the gym more often and the ability to process nutrients at faster rate, all of which will help us heal faster and allow our body to adapt to the stresses we are placing on it while working out. We want the maximum benefits with the least side effects. And this is where it gets a little tricky.

Our goal is to find the sweet spot and every human is different. With that said, the sweet spot range will be between 375mg to 750mg a week for testosterone. This will lead to a once a week injection. You can split this up into two if you want, but in my personal experience a once every five day shot of 375mg will produce all the positive effects we are looking for with virtually no side effects. At these dosages we can safely run a protocol up to 20-22 weeks with little or no side effects.

These are my recommendations from experimenting with athletes in multiple different sports and on myself. At these levels you will notice a tremendous amount of strength gains, your recovery time between workouts will be almost zero, and you will maximize your nutrient absorption and you won't feel like a pin cushion with multiple injections a week.

(Side note: we are talking only about injectable PEDs because they pass through the liver once. Meaning orals PEDs will travel through the liver twice putting more stress on your body. Most of the time when we hear about athletes who are having issues it is because orals are being taken at a high dose and causing extreme toxicity through the body.)

Deca Durabolin

Deca Durabolin was invented in the 60's and is one of the most commonly used anabolic steroids among performance enhancing athletes. It is also one of the safest. [16]

Deca provides two major benefits to the physique transformation, namely joint relief and increased nitrogen retention, promoting more nutrient absorption. Coincidentally, these are also some of the only reasons that athletes will use it. Deca is another drug that can be prescribed by a doctor and an athletic dosage, a safe dosage, would be around 200mg-400mg a week, providing all the joint relief and nutrient absorption that we could possibly need.

Human Growth Hormone (HGH)

Human Growth Hormone, used in HRT (Hormone Replacement Therapy) is produced by all living beings and and is at its highest levels in the human body during puberty.

---

[16] "Deca Durabolin." steroid.com. https://www.steroid.com/Deca-Durabolin.php. (11/2018).

Human Growth Hormone also supports the metabolism of carbohydrates, fats and minerals.[17] Unlike steroids, HGH is one of the few substances that can actually produce new muscle cells, unlike testosterone or deca durabolin which only increase the size of the cell.

HGH has been proven to not only benefit our physical form, but also produce a feeling of well being. Supplementing with HGH will promote recovery far greater than any PED we have talked about, as well as carry a pronounced positive effect on the metabolism. As it pertains to healing, HGH carries tremendous healing properties that can be beneficial to nearly all areas of the human body.[18] Some call it the fountain of youth.

With that said the real stuff is extremely expensive and degrades at a fast rate when not refrigerated. A box of HGH on the black market, if you know someone, will cost you about 500 dollars for the real stuff, Somotropin. Recently over the past ten years there has been an influx of Chinese generics, some being counterfeits and each box can go for roughly 200 bucks. Purity and quality with the generics is never guaranteed because HGH does not travel well, meaning most versions need to be refrigerated and the logistics of Chinese versions can never be guaranteed.

For the average consumer not wanting to become a professional bodybuilder and not wanting to go broke I have found doses of 2iu's to 4iu's daily to produce dramatic fat loss and muscle building results. When coupled with compounds like testosterone the effects are even greater. Meaning one compound will produce new cells, the other will grow them big-

[17] "Human Growth Hormone." steroid.com. https://www.steroid.com/Human-Growth-Hormone.php. (11/2018).

[18] "Human Growth Hormone." steroid.com. https://www.steroid.com/Human-Growth-Hormone.php. (Accessed date).

ger. HGH can be used on its own, but the effects will be much more dramatic on fat loss and muscle building when used synergistically with testosterone and/or deca together. When prescribed by a doctor, HGH will be used in conjunction with one if not both of the steroidal compounds above.

Clenbuterol Hydrochloride

Clenbuterol is a powerful bronchodilator that is used to treat breathing disorders like asthma. It is also currently illegal in the US.

For athletic training purposes clenbuterol is commonly used as a thermogenic. Clenbuterol acts by stimulating the beta-2 receptor. Beta-2 receptors are the good receptors on a fat cell that help accelerate and promote fat burning.

Clenbuterol does not actually burn fat by attacking fat cells. What it does is stimulate the metabolism by increasing the body's core temperature. Beta-2 stimulation results in the mitochondria (remember the power plants?) of the cells producing and releasing more heat. In turn, this heats up the body's temperature and enhances our metabolism. The hotter the body runs the more calories it will be burning.

Most athletes will start with 20mcg a day bumping it up 20mcg from there as needed, for as long as two weeks or until the jitters wear off. A good way to judge if you are taking too much is if you feel your central nervous system, for lack of a better term, freaking out, maybe your hands are jittery, you are not sleeping well, or you are just kind a on edge all the time, "geeking out." This would be a good indication that you are taking too much of the drug at one time and need to scale back.

A ramp up protocol is recommended because your body builds up a tolerance as far as the thermogenic effects are considered to the drug and more will have to be taken over time to achieve the fat burning results that we had earlier in the cycle.

There are a couple of theories on how long to run a clenbuterol cycle. I don't think this drug should be prevalent in many people's programs as strict nutrition and exercise will get you to where you need to go the majority of the time. However, I always keep a little on hand for when I am feeling like I am falling off the wagon, looking fluffy, and never run it for more than two to three days at a time before taking a day or two off and starting again. You shouldn't be falling off the wagon so far that you need to run clenbuterol for two weeks straight at a time. If you do that just means you have poor nutritional programing.

Side effects of PED's

Any intelligent conversation about PEDs would not be complete without the discussion of the side effects. After all, every good has some bad. Being educated on the use of each substance, their potential side effects, and how to manage them, we can negate some, if not all, of these negatives, if not get rid of them all together.

With regards to testosterone and deca durabolin we have a few concerns, not big ones, but they must still be discussed. Namely the shutdown of natural testosterone production and the increase in estrogen production. When using testosterone and even to a degree deca, what we are doing is sending a signal to the testes to stop producing testosterone. We are adding an exogenous substance which provides the same benefits that the body is producing, however in a much higher concentration. Every human will have a different sensitivity level to these compounds. Most people when using non bodybuilder dosages will have some issues - oily skin, increased estrogen production, and if you are genetically predisposed to it, hair loss, but at the dosages we are taking about there really shouldn't be any problems.

How do we negate estrogenic side effects? We take anti estrogens. Two of the most popular are Arimadex and Aromasin. For this conversation we will talk about Aromasin which is a non-steroidal aromatase inhibitor used to treat breast cancer in postmenopausal women. Both compounds are suicidal inhibitors meaning they kill your body's ability to convert testosterone and certain other drugs to estrogen.

For our journey we are going to choose Aromasin (Exemestane) to control estrogen as it is one of the newest and safest classes of breast cancer drugs out of the two and there are many studies showing that it is safe and can be used for long periods of time with virtually no side effects.[19] A dosage of 12.5 mg to 25mg every other day seems to be sufficient and depending on your sensitivity you might even be able to get away with an every three day protocol.

Restoring Natural Hormone Levels Post PED Use

At the end of your protocol you are going to want to bring your body back to normal production levels of testosterone and we have two ways to do this. The first would be to do nothing and wait for your natural production to turn back on which it inevitably will. There are pros and cons to this, one being that you will have a crash of testosterone at the end of your protocol and will have to wait longer to start feeling normal again, to start producing testosterone again in your body. The main negative of this is that most of your gains, your progress, will be lost during that time. The benefit of this method is that is literally forces your body to up regulate its testosterone receptors making them more sensitive to any

---

[19] Nabholtz, Jean-Marc A. "Long-term safety of aromatase inhibitors in the treatment of breast cancer." National Institutes of Health, U.S. National Library of Medicine. https://www.ncbi.nlm.nih.gov/pmc/articles/PMC2503653/. (12/2018).

free testosterone floating around in your body. Almost like renewing the receptors for your next protocol if you choose. You will always maintain some of your gains. The question when coming off is how much.

The smarter and more efficient method would be to tell your body to turn back on its natural testosterone production by sending a signal. We do this by taking a compound called HCG or human chorionic gonadotropin. I'm sure you have heard of the HCG diet (something we will not be discussing as even the American Medical Journal is still debating the validity of that subject).

HCG is a powerful hormone found in pregnant women and discovered in the 1920's. By administering this substance we are telling the testes to resume their natural production of testosterone in the body. This protocol is usually administered roughly around day 10 from the last dose of testosterone and for our purposes (relating to our dosages) a total of 5000mg will be administered over the next 14 days or so. An example would be 1500mg on day ten, three days later 1000mg, three days later 1000mg, three days later 1000mg, two days later 500mg. This will force the body to resume producing its natural functioning levels. I would then recommend that the person clean out for a minimum of three months before they start another protocol.

CHAPTER TWENTY TWO
In Closing

I don't want you to read this and come out with the idea that I think I am a guru or somehow know more than a doctor or your local spiritual leader. I would like you to look at me as somewhat of a journalist or record taker of sorts who has compiled, given various references, and experimented on himself, then given you a system that works for both physical and spiritual transformation. It's not the easy road, but it's a real road.

As society is getting further and further away from nature, there is an ever prevalent need for us to connect. This has led to a greater interest in self exploration, meditation, and increased personal awareness leading many people away from traditional methods of worship, religion, and self help.

I wanted to put this information into writing because it's important that if people are going to go down this road of self enlightenment, that they know it's not weird or pseudoscience. There are other people doing this. The internet is full of experts who have no face. The above text is designed to give you an idea of where you can take the limits of your personal experience with self enlightenment and physical transformation. I have not written about anything I personally have not experimented with or believe doesn't work.

My goal is to provide a base that will help you safely navigate the world of self realization and physical transformation, but the journey is yours. It is up to you to design what will work best for you. You can use some of this information, all of this information, or you can even decide to throw it all away and make your own assumptions. The only thing I request is that you do it safely and don't harm anyone else in the process. Since the dawn of humanity, inscribed on even the most ancient petroglyphs, humans have wondered what their maximum potential was and if something higher than them existed. There is no reason why we should not continue that tradition today.